Promoting Breastfeeding
Medical Settings

Edited by
Kathleen Kendall-Tackett, PhD, IBCLC, FAPA

All royalties go to the
U.S. Lactation Consultant Association.

Praeclarus Press, LLC

Praeclarus Press, LLC
2504 Sweetgum Lane
Amarillo, Texas 79124 USA
806-367-9950
www.PraeclarusPress.com

DISCLAIMER

The information contained in this publication is advisory only and is not intended to replace sound clinical judgment or individualized patient care. The author disclaims all warranties, whether expressed or implied, including any warranty as the quality, accuracy, safety, or suitability of this information for any particular purpose.

ISBN 978-1-946665-17-1

©2018. United States Lactation Consultant Association

Cover Design: Ken Tackett

Acquisition & Development: Kathleen Kendall-Tackett

Copy Editing: Chris Tackett

Layout & Design: Nelly Murariu

Contents

USLCA

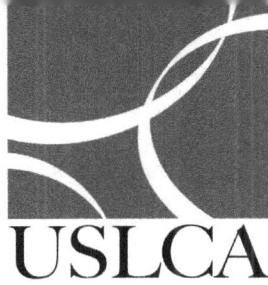

Increasing Hospital Breastfeeding Rates Through Online Education for Staff Registered Nurses

Ann Baker, DNP | Yvonne Weideman, DNP
Debra Facello, PhD

Keywords: breastfeeding, staff education, knowledge, attitude

Background: *The Baby-Friendly Hospital Initiative of 2010 recommends the proportion of mothers who breastfeed their babies in the early postpartum period should be at least 75% (Baby-Friendly USA, 2010). The exclusively breastfeeding rate at a community hospital located in the Appalachian region is 44%, well below the proposed standard. Registered nurses who lack knowledge or exhibit a negative attitude toward breastfeeding, can impede the understanding and skills necessary to empower mothers to effectively breastfeed.*

Purpose: *This performance improvement project was designed to determine whether an online educational module was effective in increasing the knowledge and improving the attitudes of nurses working with breastfeeding mothers.*

Methods: *A pre- and posttest design was used to evaluate nurse's attitudes and knowledge of breastfeeding.*

Results: *The results of the paired-sample t-test indicated a significant increase in the Breastfeeding Initiation Practice scores pre- and posttest. The exclusive breastfeeding rate had a clinically significant change from 44% to 58%.*

Conclusion: *An online educational intervention was effective in increasing the knowledge of nurses working with breastfeeding mothers. This efficient and cost-effective intervention may be valuable to hospitals desiring to increase exclusive breastfeeding rates by increasing the knowledge and skill of staff.*

Many barriers exist that inhibit the understanding and promotion of breastfeeding. A significant barrier in the support of breastfeeding is a lack of knowledge and/or negative attitudes among registered nurses (RNs) in the clinical setting. This lack of knowledge or negative attitude impedes the understanding and skills necessary for professionals to empower mothers to effectively breastfeed. Davis, Stichler, and Poeltler (2012) found that education on the benefits of breastfeeding can increase the knowledge and confidence of nurses working with breastfeeding mothers, thereby laying the foundation needed to support exclusive breastfeeding immediately following delivery of a newborn.

The Baby-Friendly Hospital Initiative of 2010 recommends that the proportion of mothers who exclusively breastfeed their babies in the early postpartum period should be at least 75% (Baby-Friendly USA, 2010). Breastfeeding has long- and short-term benefits for the mother and baby (Davis et al., 2012; Patton, Beaman, Csar, & Lewinski, 1996). The risks for mothers that do not breastfeed include increases in breast cancer, cervical cancer, postpartum depression, type 2 diabetes, and cardiovascular disease. The risks for infants who are not breastfed include an increase in obesity, gastroenteritis, leukemia, sudden infant death syndrome (SIDS), otitis media, and diabetes (Davis et al., 2012).

The exclusive breastfeeding rate at one community hospital in the Appalachian region was 44%, well below the proposed standard. Discussions with the nursing staff revealed that the staff had a lack of knowledge of breastfeeding basics and a poor attitude toward the support of exclusive breastfeeding. In an attempt to improve the exclusive breastfeeding rate at this hospital, a quality improvement project was initiated. An online educational course was used as the educational intervention and evaluated. The course was directed toward improving the nurses' knowledge, skill, and attitudes. The purpose of this article is to discuss this design, implementation, and evaluation of this quality improvement process.

A review of the literature reveals that extensive studies have been conducted on how a nurse's breastfeeding knowledge, attitudes, and skills impact exclusive breastfeeding rates. The literature suggests that educational interventions used alone for nursing staff do not influence breastfeeding rates (Fairbank et al., 2000), but when education was aimed at improving knowledge, attitude, and skills, rates were improved. This was exemplified by a study completed by Zakarija-Grkovic and Burmaz (2010), where a 20-hour United Nations Children's Fund/World Health Organization course was effective in improving breastfeeding knowledge, attitudes, and practices. In addition, a study completed by Davis et al. (2012) illustrates that teaching nurses breastfeeding basics and changing hospital policies increased breastfeeding rates. Yet another study, completed by Martens (2000), provided evidence that a 1.5-hour educational intervention was effective in increasing compliance with the Baby-Friendly Hospital Initiative, breast-feeding beliefs, and exclusive breastfeeding rates. It provided no change in breastfeeding attitudes. Although there is mixed evidence in the literature related to the ability of an educational intervention to change attitudes, there is consensus that education can improve knowledge and skills, which in turn can positively impact breastfeeding rates.

Theoretical Framework

The guiding framework for this project was Albert Bandura's Self-Efficacy Theory (see Figure 1). The © 2015 United States Lactation Consultant Association25 theory is based on the belief that individuals possess the beliefs that enable them to exercise control over thoughts, feelings, and actions that "what people think, believe, and feel affects how they behave" (Bandura, 1986). The theory states that learning occurs by attention, retention, reproduction, and motivation (Bandura, 1997). It is based on the individuals' belief in their own capabilities. There are four major sources of self-efficacy. The first is mastery experiences: performing a task successfully strengthens our self-efficacy. The second is social modeling: witnessing others successfully completing a task raises the belief in the observers' that they too can master a comparable activity. The third is social persuasion: verbal encouragement helps people overcome self-doubt and enables them to focus on task at hand. The fourth is psychological responses: minimizing stress and elevating mood can improve self-efficacy (Bandura, 1992).

Bandura's theory supports the use of an online educational learning environment without distractions, nurse's ability to retain the information provided, opportunities to perform techniques successfully, and motivation through positive feedback and support (Bandura, 1997). All four major sources of self-efficacy were incorporated in this performance improvement project. The intervention provided nurses with information to increase knowledge, reproduce learned information through experiences, verbal praise, guidance, and resources that helped reduce stress.

Method

The project was reviewed and approved by the human subject review committee at the community hospital and by the university's internal review board (Pittsburgh, Pennsylvania) prior to data collection. Twenty RNs who work in the neonatal unit located in the Appalachian region were invited to participate. A meeting was organized to explain the quality improvement project and the related goals. Consents were also obtained at that time. Eighteen of the 20 RNs consented to participate in the performance improvement project. Although each nurse was required to complete the mandatory education, only the data from those nurses who elected to participate was used in the analysis.

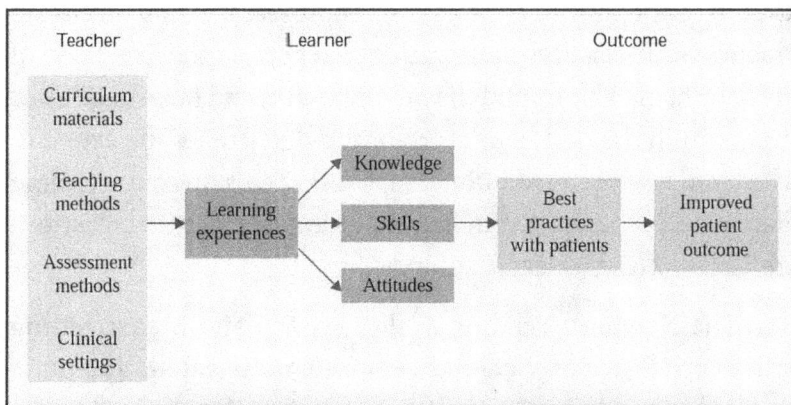

Figure 1. Bandura's Self-Efficacy Theory

Measures

Prior to completing the educational intervention, assessment of breastfeeding knowledge level and attitude toward exclusive breastfeeding was conducted through the use of the Newborn Feeding Ability Questionnaire (Appendix A), the Breastfeeding Initiation Practice Scale (Appendix B), and the Breastfeeding Attitude Questionnaire (Appendix C).

The Newborn Feeding Ability Questionnaire has 21 items with responses on a 5-point Likert scale. The Newborn Feeding Ability has a possible total score of 105 with higher scores reflecting greater knowledge. The items assess three areas. The first area is knowledge about physiological and emotional benefits of skin-to-skin contact for the newborn and mother. The second area is knowledge of indicators of effective suckling and milk transfer. The third area assesses work practices that interfere with newborn feeding ability.

The Breastfeeding Initiation Practice Scale has 12 items and uses case scenarios involving commonly observed birthing room events with items rated on a 5-point Likert scale. The highest possible score is 60, with higher scores reflecting better practice (Creedy, Cantrill, & Cooke, 2008). The Breastfeeding Initiation Practice Scale requires participants to report on the likelihood of the baby being able to find the nipple, attach, and breastfeed effectively within the first hour of birth, and determines the extent to which nurses promoted uninterrupted skin-to-skin contact immediately after birth and promoted baby's innate ability to breastfeed are assessed (Creedy et al., 2008).

The Newborn Feeding Ability (a5 .87) and Breastfeeding Initiation Practice Scale (a5 .74) demonstrated adequate internal consistency. Construct validity was determined by the use of exploratory factor analyses (Creedy et al., 2008). Criterion validity was drawn from a critical review of literature on breastfeeding initiation and expert review (Creedy et al., 2008). Predictive validity for the Newborn Feeding Ability scores contributed to 31.5% of variance in reported practice, which indicated moderate predictive validity (Creedy et al., 2008). The author received permission to use the Newborn Feeding Questionnaire and the Breastfeeding Initiation Practice Scale prior the to start of the project by contacting Biomed Central Open Access license agreement.

The Breastfeeding Attitude Questionnaire is an 11-item survey with items rated on a 5-point Likert scale. The highest possible score of the Breastfeeding Attitude Scale is 55. The higher the score, the more positive the nurses' attitude is regarding breastfeeding (Martens, 2000). The tool demonstrated test–retest reliability over a 1-week period, with nonsignificant differences using paired t test and highly significant Pearson's correlation coefficients (r5 .9, p, .001). The Breastfeeding Attitude tool was considered internally consistent, with Cronbach's alpha scores of .92, .92, and .95, respectively, during the pilot test and .84, .86, and .89 during the actual research (Martens, 2000). The permission to the Breastfeeding Attitude Scale was received from SAGE Copyright Clearance Center. Thus, the Newborn Feeding Ability, Breastfeeding Initiation Practice Scale, and Breastfeeding Attitude Questionnaire are valid and reliable tools for the assessment of knowledge, practice, and attitude of nurses toward breastfeeding.

Procedure

The consenting nurses completed the questionnaires in a private area of the nursing unit via paper and pencil. To ensure confidentiality, envelopes were provided for the completed questionnaires and a locked box was located in a private area for completed questionnaires. Once the nurses completed the questionnaires, education was provided through an online self-directed learning module. The module was located on the health stream network and developed by Lippincott Williams and Wilkins. HealthStream (2012) is the electronic database of preselected educational modules for the hospital. The module titled Breast-feeding Assistance was selected for the intervention. It took approximately 30–40 minutes to complete.

The module reviewed breastfeeding positions, breast care for new mothers, special considerations, complications, and documentation. The module was designed to increase knowledge of positions, techniques, and common problems associated with teaching a new mother to exclusively breastfeed her infant. Four weeks following the conclusion of the online educational module, the RNs again completed the Newborn Feeding Ability, Breastfeeding Initiation Practice Scale, and Breastfeeding Attitude Questionnaire.

Envelopes were then provided for completed questionnaires and a locked box was located in a private area for completed questionnaires to ensure confidentiality. To assess exclusive breastfeeding rate changes, the exclusive breastfeeding rates were recorded prior to the online educational model and following completion.

Results

Individual responses from each participant were aggregated in two phases: pretest (n5 18) and posttest (n5 18). The breastfeeding rate was collected prior to initiation and again 4 weeks following completion of the educational model. All data was deidentified and analyzed using the statistical analysis program SPSS 16. All results were normally distributed and parametric procedures were used.

Nursing knowledge related to observing pre-feeding behavior, mother/baby care, attachment, and positioning practices were measured through the Breastfeeding Initiation Practice Scale. There was statistically significant differences in t-test scores between the pretest scores (M5 38.611, SD5 7.883) and the posttest scores (M5 42.222, SD5 5.956) with p5.007 with CI 5 95. Pre- and post-Cronbach's alpha scores were .84 and .75 for the Breastfeeding Initiation Practice Scale, thus indicating it was a reliable measure.

Knowledge of skin-to-skin contact, physiological stability, newborn innate abilities, work practices, and effective breast-feeding were measured pre- and posttest through the Newborn Feeding Ability Questionnaire. The attitudes of the nurses were measured pre- and posttest using the Breastfeeding Attitude Questionnaire. There were no statistically significant differences in either of the questionnaires results. The hospital's pre- and post-online educational module breastfeeding rates were 44% and 58%, thus demonstrating a statistically significant increase of 14% (p5 .007). The increase was clinically significant because of the impact on the health of the mother and baby.

Discussion

The findings of this performance improvement project suggest that increasing the RNs knowledge relating to observing pre-feeding behavior, mother/baby care, attachment, and positioning practices contributes to increased breastfeeding rates. This is in contrast to the findings of Fairbank et al. (2000). However, it is comparable to the findings of Davis et al. (2012) and Martens (2000), in that online education improves hospital breastfeeding rates. The findings support Albert Bandura's Self-Efficacy Theory, in that learning occurs by attention, retention, reproduction, and motivation (Bandura, 1997). The

Breastfeeding Initiation Practice Scale showed significant differences in pre and post educational scores. Nursing knowledge related to observing pre-feeding behavior, mother/baby care, attachment, and positioning practices were measured and showed an increase. This online educational intervention is effective in increasing knowledge and breastfeeding rates, as shown by the 14% increase. To sustain the positive change noted in this project, the policy is being modified to require that all RNs receive mandatory education every 3 months.

The Newborn Feeding Ability Questionnaire measured the nurses' knowledge of skin-to-skin contact, physiological stability, and newborn innate abilities relating to work practices and effective breastfeeding showed no significant changes between pre- and posttest. This is most likely because of the fact that the educational module discussed basic breastfeeding issues rather than the items measured by the Newborn Feeding Ability Questionnaire. Education relating to these issues might further increase the exclusively breastfeeding rate.

The Breastfeeding Attitude Scale showed no statically significant results. The initial discussions with the nurses revealed a poor attitude toward breastfeeding. However, this may not have been accurate because the nurses' scores on the Breastfeeding Attitude Scale did not show a poor attitude with mean score of 45.45 out of a possible 55. It is possible that the lack of knowledge led to a sense of frustration that was perceived by the interviewers as a poor attitude versus an unwillingness to promote breastfeeding which was measured by the Breastfeeding Attitude Scale.

The exclusively breastfeeding rate showed an increase of 14% 4 weeks after the intervention. Although the increase was not enough to enable the hospital to achieve the Baby-Friendly Initiative benchmark of 75%, it was statistically significant. The increase was significant because 14% more new mothers who received support from the nurses could be expected to decrease their risk of breast cancer, cervical cancer, postpartum depression, type 2 diabetes, and cardiovascular disease associated with exclusively breastfeeding. In addition, 14% more babies will have a decreased risk for obesity, gastroenteritis, leukemia, SIDS, otitis media, and diabetes because of being exclusively breastfed.

The project was significant to the hospital in that it reinforced the benefits of exclusively breastfeeding and enhanced the knowledge of the importance of exclusively breastfeeding to administration, management, and RNs. Following the performance improvement project, the hospital implemented a breastfeeding committee. The committee reviewed the breastfeeding policies and determined major revisions were needed. Policy revision of the breastfeeding policies heightened the awareness and the importance of exclusive breastfeeding. In addition to improving the nurses' knowledge, the online educational intervention was cost-effective and had had minimal implementation time and effort. Its success in improving exclusive breastfeeding rates led the hospital to mandate breastfeeding education for the RNs, and it is hoped that continuation of breastfeeding education will increase the rate to meet the recommended benchmark. Different online modules will be completed every 3 months. Nursing needs will be evaluated every 3 months by use of surveys, and evaluation of the exclusive breastfeeding rate will be collected monthly.

Thirteen of the 18 participants had obtained a bachelor's degree in nursing and 5 of the 18 had obtained an associate degree in nursing. They all had worked in the nursery for at least 3 years, and 10 of the 18 had previously breastfed at least one child. Suggestions for further research include assessing the impact of the RN's length of employment, educational level, and prior breastfeeding experience on breastfeeding knowledge, skill, attitude, and associated breastfeeding rates. Other types of online educational interventions should be assessed and their impact on exclusive breastfeeding should also be investigated.

Conclusion

This performance improvement project was designed to determine the effectiveness of an online educational module on the knowledge and attitudes toward exclusive breastfeeding and subsequent impact on exclusive breastfeeding rates. Although the project was limited in that it involved a limited convenience sample, it demonstrated the value of online education for nurses to significantly impact their knowledge and improve exclusive breastfeeding rates at a small hospital in the Appalachian region. Because exclusive breastfeeding has many benefits for the health and well-being of mother and baby, online educational courses similar to this can lead to increased exclusively breastfeeding rates. This result is significant for those working in maternal child nursing and for those institutions desiring to improve their exclusively breastfeeding rate to meet the Baby-Friendly Initiatives.

References

Baby-Friendly USA. (2010). *Guidelines and evaluation criteria for facilities seeking baby-friendly designation.* Sandwich, MA: Author. Retrieved from http://www.babyfriendlyusa.org/eng/docs/2010_Guidelines_Criteria_4.19.11.pdf

Bandura, A. (1986). *Social foundations of thought and action: A social cognitive theory.* New York, NY: Prentice Hall.

Bandura, A. (1992). Exercise of personal agency through the self-efficacy mechanisms. In R. Schwarzer (Ed.), *Self-efficacy:*

Thought control of action (pp. 3–38). Washington, DC: Hemisphere. Bandura, A. (1997). *Self-efficacy. The exercise of control.* New York, NY: Freeman.

Creedy, D., Cantrill, R., & Cooke, M. (2008). Assessing midwives' breastfeeding knowledge: Properties of the newborn feeding ability questionnaire and breastfeeding initiation practices scale. *International Breastfeeding Journal, 3,* 7. Retrieved from http://www.internationalbreastfeedingjournal.com/content/3/1/7

Davis, S., Stichler, J., & Poeltler, D. (2012). Increasing exclusive breastfeeding rates in the well-baby population: An evidence-based changed project. *Nursing for Women's Health, 16*(6), 461–470. http://dx.doi.org/10.111/j.1751-486X.2012.01774.x

Fairbank, L., O'Meara, S., Renfrew, M., Woolridge, M., Sowden, A., & Lister-Sharp, D. (2000). A systematic review to evaluate the effectiveness of interventions to promote the initiation of breastfeeding. *Health Technology Assessment, 4*(25), 1–171.

HealthStream. (2012). *Breast-feeding assistance.* Philadelphia, PA: Lippincott Williams & Wilkins.

Martens, P. J. (2000). Does breastfeeding education affect nursing staff beliefs, exclusive breastfeeding rates, and Baby-Friendly Hospital Initiative compliance? The experience of a small, rural Canadian hospital. *Journal of Human Lactation, 16*(4), 309–318. http://dx.doi.org/10.1177/089033440001600407

Patton, C., Beaman, M., Csar, N., & Lewinski, C. (1996). Nurses' attitudes and behaviors that promote breastfeeding. *Journal of Human Lactation, 12*(2), 111–115. http://dx.doi.org/10.1177/089033449601200213

Zakarija-Grkovic, I., & Burmaz, T. (2010). Effectiveness of the UNICEF/WHO 20-hour course in improving health professionals' knowledge, practices, and attitudes to breastfeeding: Before/after study of 5 maternity facilities in Croatia. *Croatia Medical Journal, 51,* 396–405. http://dx.doi.org/10.3325/cmj.2010.51.396

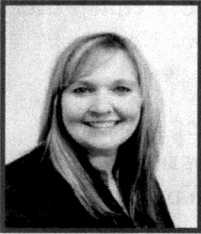

Ann Baker, DNP, is currently the chair of the Nursing Department at Wheeling Jesuit University in Wheeling, West Virginia. She is also an assistant professor of nursing within the program. Dr. Baker earned her doctor of nursing practice from Duquesne University, her master's in nursing from Wheeling Jesuit University and her bachelor of science in nursing from Wheeling Jesuit University. Dr. Baker is also an International Board Certified Lactation Consultant. Dr. Baker's scholarship has emerged from her clinical expertise, passion to educate others, and aspiration to promote health and well-being within the community. Dr. Baker has worked in various clinical settings and developed a passion for maternal child health nursing. Dr. Baker is currently completing her family nurse practitioner certification at Franciscan University of Steubenville.

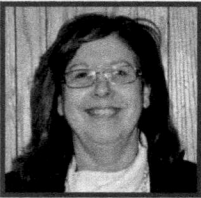

Yvonne Weideman, DNP, is assistant professor at Duquesne University. Dr. Weideman earned her doctor of nursing practice from Duquesne University, her Master of Business Administration from Robert Morris University and her bachelor of science in nursing from Duquesne University. Dr. Weideman's scholarship has emerged through the intersection of her clinical expertise, passion for nursing education, and desire to positively impact the health of communities and the people residing in them. It has included a patent for a virtual pregnancy and the design, implementation, and evaluation of a virtual clinic where students learn maternity and newborn concepts and multiple national presentations centered on service learning, community–academic partnerships, simulation, and interprofessional education.

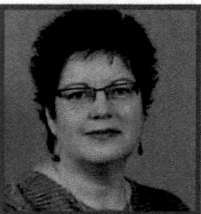

Debra Facello, PhD, began her career as a nurse in 1975 as an associate degree in nursing graduate of Clarion University. In 1978, she earned a bachelor of science in nursing from West Liberty State College and completed a teaching certification in Health K-12. It was in 1982 that she earned her master's degree in nursing and in 2008, earned a PhD in nursing from West Virginia

University. Debra began teaching nursing in March of 1979 at Ohio Valley Hospital School of Nursing in Steubenville, Ohio. She later moved to faculty positions at the university level, specializing in maternal/newborn nursing. She currently serves as the director of the Master of Science in Nursing program at Franciscan University of Steubenville in Steubenville, Ohio.

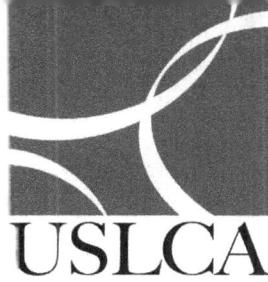

Pilot Study of Breastfeeding Support on the Night Shift

Betsy Ayers, BSN, RN, IBCLC, RLC

Jane Grassley, PhD, RN, IBCLC, RLC

Kristen Koprowski, BSN, RN

Keywords: breastfeeding support, nurses, night shift, exclusive breastfeeding

Exclusive breastfeeding during the first 6 months of life facilitates optimal health for mothers and their infants and is a hospital discharge perinatal core measure. The purpose of this study was to identify nurses' experiences, perceptions, and practices of breastfeeding support on the night shift, recognize barriers, and offer recommendations to maintain exclusive initial breastfeeding. Data were collected using an anonymous 14-item online questionnaire, developed from the literature. The results identified babies' behavior and maternal fatigue as the biggest challenges to breastfeeding support on the night shift. Our recommendations include education of families regarding normal nighttime behaviors and encouragement of mothers to nap when their newborn is napping. More research is needed with a larger, national, and more geographically representative sample to validate these findings.

Exclusive breastfeeding is a challenging goal for hospital staff. Organizations, such as the Centers for Disease Control and Prevention (2014) in the United States, and the World Health Organization (2014), have established exclusive breastfeeding in the first 6 months as the gold standard. Exclusive Breast Milk Feeding (PC-05a) is one of the newest quality measures for The Joint Commission (2014), which accredits hospitals in the United States. One of the breastfeeding goals of the Healthy People 2020 is to reduce the proportion of breastfeeding newborns who receive infant formula within the first 2 days of life from 24.2% (currently) to 14.2%, and support a second goal of 46.2% exclusive breastfeeding during the first 3 months (U.S. Department of Health and Human Services, 2014).

Staff giving supplements to newborns was one of three hospital practices that negatively influences exclusive breastfeeding (DeClercq, Labbok, Sakala, & O'Hara, 2009). According to Howard et al. (2003), the most significant predictor of breastfeeding duration was supplementation of breastfeeding while in the hospital. Early supplementation can potentially impact a newborn's health. For example, breastfed newborns carry a more stable and uniform microflora population in their guts when compared to those fed infant formula, which decreases their risk of gastrointestinal illness (Bezirtzoglou, Tsiotsias, & Welling, 2011). Scientists demonstrated 15 years ago that relatively small amounts of formula supplementation of breastfed infants will result in shifts from a breastfed to a formula-fed pattern microbiota (Mackie, Sghir, & Gaskins, 1999).

Understanding the factors associated with supplementation of healthy breastfeeding newborns before hospital discharge is imperative to supporting exclusive breastfeeding. Several studies have identified the hospital night shift as a barrier to exclusive breastfeeding. In their study of factors associated with in-hospital formula supplementation of healthy breastfeeding newborns, Gagnon, Leduc, Waghorn, Yang, and Platt (2005) found that newborns were most at risk for supplementation between 7:00 p.m. and 9:00 a.m. Being born at night, or staying a second night, increased the odds of supplementation with infant formula in another study (Grassley, Schleis, Bennett, Chapman, & Lind, 2014). The breastfeeding beliefs and practices of the night shift staff may contribute to increased formula supplementation at night. Using qualitative methods, researchers identified that nurses on the night shift tended to place a mother's need for rest while in the hospital at a higher priority than the negative impact of formula supplementation on breastfeeding (Nickel, Taylor, Labbok, Weiner, & Williamson, 2013; Weddig, Baker, & Auld, 2011). Evidence suggests that the risk for supplementation increases the second night because newborns are typically more awake, tend to cluster feed (DaMota, Bañuelos, Goldbronn, Vera-Beccera, & Heinig, 2012), and mothers are more fatigued (Cloherty, Alexander, & Holloway, 2004).

Despite the importance of the night shift as a barrier to exclusive breastfeeding before hospital discharge, few studies have been conducted to study this phenomenon. Therefore, the purpose of this pilot study was to explore nurses' perceptions of the barriers to breastfeeding support encountered during the night shift and offer recommendations to maintain exclusive initial breastfeeding.

Methods

Study Design

This study used a descriptive survey design. Because an appropriate instrument was not available within the literature, the researchers developed a 14-item questionnaire to determine challenges to breastfeeding support and resources needed on the night shift using their experience as International Board Certified Lactation Consultants (IBCLCs) and the literature (Dennis, 2006; Morrison & Ludington-Hoe, 2012; Parry, Ip, Chau, Wu, & Tarrant, 2013; Tender et al., 2009). The survey of breastfeeding support on the night shift was thus designed to assess breastfeeding support on the night shift, patterns of infant behavior/health, and maternal health and knowledge that may undermine exclusive breastfeeding in the first days after birth. The questionnaire also encouraged nurses to provide suggestions for resources that would improve exclusive breastfeeding on the night shift. All but two questions were multiple-choice; and some allowed for multiple answers. Two questions asked for an open-ended response: "What do you do when a breastfeeding mom asks for formula for newborn?" and "What can be done during day shift to better prepare mothers for breastfeeding on night shift?"

Data Collection

The hospital system's institutional ethics review board. The questionnaire was placed online and a recruitment flyer for this study was distributed to 29 night shift nursing staff during the Fall 2013 staff meeting. In addition, a recruitment email explaining the study was sent to all night nursing staff with a link to the online study survey. A follow-up reminder email was sent approximately 1 month later. Potential participants were given the opportunity to ask questions at the staff meeting or via email. To keep responses anonymous, a waiver of documentation of consent was requested. An informational sheet containing the elements of informed consent was presented to participants, with completion of the questionnaire signifying consent.

Setting and Sample

The study sample consisted of 24 registered nurses and 5 non-nurse clinical assistant personnel (CAPs) supporting labor/delivery and mother/baby units. All participants worked the night shift at a Level 2 suburban hospital located in the Mountain West, having 1,200 births per year. The study institution had a current exclusive breastfeeding rate of 75% and a formula supplementation rate of about 25%.

Data Analysis

Study data and the online questionnaire were collected and managed using Research Electronic Data Capture (REDCap) hosted by the Institute of Translational Health Science, supported by grant UL1RR025014 from the National Center for Research Resources/National Institutes of Health at the University of Washington. REDCap is a secure, web-based application designed to support data capture for research studies (Harris et al., 2009). Data were analyzed using SAS. Descriptive statistics were used to answer the research question.

Results

The majority (17 out of 29) of night shift staff completed the online questionnaire for a return rate of 59%. The study results tell a story of the unique challenges nursing staff face when promoting exclusive breastfeeding on the night shift (see Tables 1 and 2). The dynamics of newborn health and behavior were the main challenges to exclusive breastfeeding identified by study participants. The nursing staff ranked infant health as the main reason a newborn may receive formula before hospital discharge, followed by breastfeeding and/or latch problems. Infant behavior was most often identified as their major challenge when providing breastfeeding support (41.2%). According to our results, most of the respondents listed hunger as the top reason a newborn cries in the first 48 hours of birth (60%).

Mother/infant dyads having a breastfeeding problem, such as trouble latching, was the second ranked reason given for formula supplementation. However, when encountering breastfeeding problems, offering formula was not their first action; 67% of participants teach feeding cues and assist with latching the newborn, which they reported most often as taking the most time (70%). Although the majority of nursing staff had 2 or more years of working on this maternity unit, and 94% said they were extremely or moderately comfortable with breastfeeding support, 24% reported a need for an IBCLC on the night shift. Additionally, when asked for recommendations and resources needed that would improve breastfeeding, 73% participants ranked having an IBCLC on their shift as the number one most-needed resource (73%).

The resources most often used by nurses were another nurse/CAP (94%) or the parent resource booklet (47%). The parent resource booklet is an educational booklet that instructs parents on normal newborn behaviors and teaches mothers how to care for themselves after the baby is born. Several staff recommended that mothers be encouraged to take naps in 2-hour blocks during the day, particularly when their infants are sleeping. Education about newborn nighttime feeding behaviors, such as cluster feeding, taught during early labor was also suggested. Study participants also advocated that IBCLCs during the day shift should see all breastfeeding mothers at least once before discharge. According to our results, the middle of the 12-hour night shift, 11:00 p.m. to 3:00 a.m., was reported to be the most challenging time (53%), whereas earlier in the shift, 7:00 p.m. to 11:00 p.m., and later in the shift, 3:00 a.m. to 7:00 a.m., were evenly divided at approximately 24%.

Table 1. Challenges and Resources Needed to Support Breastfeeding on the Night Shift	
Response Options by Item	%
Takes RN the most time when helping mom breastfeed	
Placing baby skin to skin	0
Calming baby before feed	0
Settling baby after feed	0
Positioning mom and/or baby for feed	70.0
Discussion with/teaching parents about feed	30.0
Time of night most challenging	
7:00 p.m. to 11:00 p.m.	23.5
11:00 p.m. to 3:00 a.m.	52.9
3:00 a.m. to 7:00 a.m.	23.5
Resources RN has used to help with breastfeeding[a]	
None	0
"Baby's first month" booklet	47.1
Another RN or CAP	94.1
Website(s)	0
Other (responses included book, person outside organization)	17.6
Comfort level of RN in helping a mother breastfeed	
Extremely	41.2
Moderately	52.9
Slightly	0
Not at all	6.0
Biggest challenge for RN in providing breastfeeding support on night shift	
Mom is too tired or sick	11.8
Baby's behavior	41.2
No dedicated lactation nurse	23.5
Nurse/couplet ratio	17.6
Nurse experience with breastfeeding	0
Other (responses: need more education)	5.9
RN first response when baby would not settle/will no longer latch according to mother	
Offer to take baby to nursery so mom can sleep	6.7
Teach mom about feeding cues and assist with relatching	66.7
Offer formula	0
Encourage mom to pump or hand express for spoon or cup feed	0
Demonstrate 5s	26.7
RN perception of main reason a newborn cries in the first 48 hours	
Wet/dirty diaper	20.0
Hunger	60.0
Cold/hot	0
Not being held/touched/swaddled	13.3
Pain	6.7
Other	0
RN perception of resources needed at night to support breastfeeding[a]	
Script for education regarding supplementation	20.0
RN/CAP education regarding normal newborn night behavior	20.0
Opportunity to shadow lactation consultant	20.0
Designated lactation nurse on night shift	73.3
Access to breastfeeding manual/book	26.7
Other (responses: repeat shadow/more education with lactation consultant)	20.0

Note. CAP = clinical assistant personnel; RN = registered nurse.

[a]Multiple answers allowed.

Response Options by Item	Rank 1 = least common 10 = most common
Table 2. Registered Nurse (RN) Perceptions of Reasons for Supplementation on Night Shift	
RN perception of main reasons newborns are supplemented while in hospital	
Infant's health (i.e., hypoglycemia, jaundice, extreme weight loss)	6.7
Breastfeeding/latch problem	6.7
Maternal fatigue	5.6
Believed insufficient milk supply/colostrum	5.5
Unexpected frequent feedings during expected hours of sleep	5.4
Maternal health (i.e., cesarean birth, hemorrhage, IV magnesium)	4.8
Baby's doctor order/suggestion	4.3
Pressure from outside (i.e., nurse, family)	3.5
OB doctor suggestion	2.0
RN perception of factors associated with infant's health/behavior that increases supplementation during night shift	
Hypoglycemia	8.0
Extreme weight loss (i.e., more than 10%)	6.4
Excessive crying during expected hours of sleep	5.8
Jaundice	5.2
Tight jaw or not bringing tongue over gum line	4.4
Excessive sleepiness in baby; not rooting, and so forth	3.8
NICU admission to rule out sepsis	3.5
Vacuum or forceps birth	3.1
Respiratory distress	2.3
Circumcision (males)	2.3
RN perception of factors associated with mother's health/knowledge that increases supplementation during night shift	
Lack of knowledge of baby's normal sleep and feeding patterns (i.e., cluster feeding more common on second night)	6.8
Fatigue	6.4
Painful and/or difficulty latching	5.8
Lack of knowledge of small newborn stomach	5.1
Lack of knowledge of normal amount of colostrum	5.7
Birth complication, hemorrhage, retained placenta, IV magnesium after birth	4.9
Caesarean birth	3.6
History of breast surgery (i.e., reduction, implants)	2.9
OB doctor ordered sleeping medication	2.2
Hormonal imbalance (i.e., thyroid, polycystic ovary syndrome)	1.9

Note. IV = intravenous; NICU = neonatal intensive care unit; OB = obstetrics.

Discussion

This pilot study is particularly important because it is one of the few studies asking nurses on the night shift their impressions of the barriers they encounter to promoting exclusive breast-feeding and offering breastfeeding support. As in other studies, infant health (e.g., blood glucose) and behavior were primary reasons for supplementation (DaMota et al., 2012; Gagnon et al., 2005). Participants identified maternal fatigue as the second most common reason for supplementation, which is consistent with Cloherty et al. (2004) and Gagnon et al. (2005). Participants ranked mothers' method of birth as an uncommon reason for supplementation, which differs from findings reported in other studies, which identify infants who experience a cesarean birth as having the highest rate of supplementation (Parry et al., 2013).

The study has limitations. One limitation of this pilot study is that no survey question identified a newborn's location during the night as a factor (i.e., newborn nursery vs. mother's room). Another limitation is the size of the sample. A larger study is planned in which the survey would be distributed through a professional nursing organization. A final limitation is that the study setting does not have a Baby-Friendly Hospital Initiative (BFHI) designation, which can affect nurses' attitudes and breastfeeding support practices, particularly on nights. Weddig et al. (2011) reported that nurses working nights in a BFHI-designated hospital were more likely to encourage 24-hour rooming-in for the mother/infant dyad and less likely to provide formula supplementation than those working in a non–BFHI-designated facility.

Clinical Implications

These study findings have clinical relevance for IBCLCs as well as mother/baby nurses working in hospital settings. First, there is a need for nurses and parents to understand expected newborn behavior in the first 48 hours after birth. The majority (60%) of participants listed hunger as the top reason a newborn cries in the first 48 hours after birth. They also reported that mothers' lack of knowledge related to cluster feedings on the second night increased the rate of supplementation. Both of these responses are indicative of a common belief that an awake and/or crying newborn is hungry. The normal, frequent feedings on the second night are interpreted as a mother not having enough milk to satisfy her newborn (DaMota et al., 2012). Nurses may also interpret this expected newborn behavior as hunger and offer formula (Gagnon et al., 2005). This is at odds with the small size of a newborn's stomach, which normally holds only 6 to 12 ml of fluid, during the first 48 hours of life (Santoro, Martinez, Ricco, & Jorge, 2010). An infant's crying can stem from many reasons, such as hunger or simply the desire to be held. Bergman, an expert in kangaroo care—the practice of keeping mothers and their infants skin-to-skin as often as possible, teaches that humans have a biological need for togetherness (Spangjer, 2001). According to Bergman, human infants are the most immature of all mammals at birth; they need to be fed frequently and thrive best when held skin to skin against their mother's body (Spangjer, 2001). A newborn learns to trust its caregiver based on the caregivers responsiveness to their cries (Narvaez, 2012).

To counter this belief, both nurses and parents can be taught about what to expect with normal newborn behavior, as well as the importance to infants of staying close to their mothers. Patient education can better prepare mothers for what to expect their second night in the hospital. Nurses can help parents recognize hunger cues and understand that their infants will be more wakeful and need to feed more often the second night. To mitigate maternal fatigue and prepare for the more wakeful second night, IBCLCs, as well as nurses can encourage mothers to take naps and rest while their newborn is sleeping during the day. This may also mean limiting visiting hours.

The majority of nurses (93%) in this study indicated that they were either moderately or extremely comfortable helping mother's breastfeed. However, the top resource requested was an IBCLC on the night shift. A possible reason for this finding is that providing breastfeeding support, particularly of a mother/newborn dyad having difficulties, may compete with the nurses' ability to adequately care for their other patients. Nickel et al. (2013) identified that hospitals rely heavily on IBCLCs to provide breastfeeding support. The role of this resource requires further study in relationship-to-work load on the night shift.

Conclusion

The night shift presents unique challenges to exclusive breast-feeding particularly related to expectations of newborn behavior and maternal fatigue. Strategies for teaching parents and health-care professionals about normal newborn breastfeeding behavior, and how to prepare for the wakefulness of the second night, need to be developed. Further study is needed to determine if the presence of a designated lactation professional on the night shift is essential to promoting exclusive breastfeeding before hospital discharge.

Acknowledgments: The authors wish to thank all of the night shift staff that responded to the survey and the directors of the participating units. The authors would also like to acknowledge the Center for Nursing Excellence and the Operation Innovation Writing Workshop within our organization, and the University of Washington, for REDCap data support (UI RR025014 from NCRR/NIH) prepare for the wakefulness of the second night, need to be developed. Further study is needed to determine if the presence of a desig-nated lactation professional on the night shift is essential to promoting exclusive breastfeeding before hospital discharge.

References

Bezirtzoglou, E., Tsiotsias, A., & Welling, G. W. (2011). Microbiota profile in feces of breast-and formula-fed newborns by using fluorescence in situ hybridization (FISH). *Anaerobe, 17*, 478–482. http://dx.doi.org/10.1016/j.anaerobe.2011.03.009

Centers for Disease Control and Prevention. (2014). *Breastfeeding report card 2014.* Retrieved from http://www.cdc.gov/breastfeeding/data/reportcard.htm

Cloherty, M., Alexander, J., & Holloway, I. (2004). Supplementing breast-fed babies in the UK to protect their mothers from tiredness or distress. *Midwifery, 20*(2), 194–204. http://dx.doi.org/10.1016/j.midw.2003.09.002

DaMota, K., Bañuelos, J., Goldbronn, J., Vera-Beccera, L., & Heinig, J. (2012). Maternal request for in-hospital supplementation of healthy breastfed infants among low-income women. *Journal of Human Lactation, 28*(4), 476–482. http://dx.doi.org/10.1177/0890334412445299

DeClercq, E., Labbok, M., Sakala, C., & O'Hara, M. (2009). Hospitals practices and women's likelihood of fulfilling their intention to exclusively breastfeed. *American Journal of Public Health, 99*(5), 929–935.

Dennis, C. L. (2006). Identifying predictors of breastfeeding self-efficacy in the immediate postpartum period. *Research in Nursing and Health, 29,* 256–268.

Gagnon, A. J., Leduc, G., Waghorn, K., Yang, H., & Platt, R. W. (2005). In-hospital supplementation of healthy breastfeeding newborns. *Journal of Human Lactation, 21*(4), 397–405.

Grassley, J. S., Schleis, J., Bennett, S., Chapman, S., & Lind, B. (2014). Reasons for initial formula supplementation of healthy breastfeeding newborns. *Nursing for Women's Health, 18,* 196–203. http://dx.doi.org/10.1111/1751-486X.12120

Harris, P. A., Taylor, R., Thielke, R., Payne, J., Gonzalez, N., & Conde, J. G. (2009). Research electronic data capture (REDCap)—A metadata-driven methodology and workflow process for providing translational research informatics support. *Journal of Biomedical Informatics, 42*(2), 377–381.

Howard, C. R., Howard, F. M., Lanphear, B., Eberly, S., deBlieck, E. A., Oakes, D., & Lawrence, R. A. (2003). Randomized clinical trial of pacifier use and bottle-feeding or cupfeeding and their effect on breastfeeding. *Pediatrics, 111*(3), 511–518. http://dx.doi.org/10.1542/peds.111.3.511

Mackie, R. I., Sghir A., & Gaskins H. R. (1999). Developmental microbial ecology of the neonatal gastrointestinal tract. *American Journal of Clinical Nutrition, 69*(5), 1035S–1045S.

Morrison, B., & Ludington-Hoe, S. (2012) Interruptions to breastfeeding dyads in an LDRP unit. *American Journal of Maternal Child Nursing, 37*(1), 36–41.

Narvaez, D. (2012). Dangers of "Crying it out": Damaging children and their relationships for the long-term. *Clinical Lactation, 3*(1), 32–35.

Nickel, N. C., Taylor, E. C., Labbok, M. H., Weiner, B. J., & Williamson, N. E. (2013). Applying organisation theory to understand barriers and facilitators to the implementation of baby-friendly: A multisite qualitative study. *Midwifery, 29,* 956–964. http://dx.doi.org/10.1016/j.midw.2012.12.001

Parry, J. E., Ip, D. K., Chau, P. Y., Wu, K. M., & Tarrant, M. (2013). Predictors and consequences of in-hospital formula supplementation for healthy breastfeeding newborns. *Journal of Human Lactation, 29*(4), 527–536. http://dx.doi.org/10.1177/ 0890334413474719

Santoro, W., Jr., Martinez, F. E., Ricco, R. G., & Jorge, S. M., (2010). Colostrum ingested during the first day of life by exclusively breastfed healthy newborn infants. *Journal of Pediatrics, 156*(1), 29–32. http://dx.doi.org/10.1016/j.jpeds .2009.07.009

Spangjer, P. (2001). Kangaroo mother care. *New Beginnings, 18*(5),178.

Tender, J. A., Janakiram, J., Arce, E., Mason, R., Jordan, T., Marsh, J., . . . Moon, R. Y. (2009). Reasons for in-hospital formula supplementation of breastfed infants from low-income families. *Journal of Human Lactation, 25*(1) 11–17.

The Joint Commission. (2014). *National quality measures.* Retrieved from https://manual.jointcommission.org/releases/TJC2014A1/ MIF0170.html

U.S. Department of Health and Human Services. (2014). *Healthy people 2020.* Retrieved from https://www.healthypeople.gov/Weddig, J., Baker, S. S., & Auld, G. (2011). Perspectives of hospital-based nurses on breastfeeding initiation best practices. *Journal of Obstetric, Gynecologic, & Neonatal Nursing, 40*(2), 166–178. http://dx.doi.org/10.1111/j.1552-6909.2011.01232.x

World Health Organization. (2014). *10 facts on breastfeeding.* Retrieved from http://www.who.int/features/factfilies/breastfeeding/en/

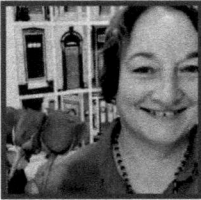

Betsy Ayers, BSN, RN, IBCLC, RLC, is a practicing lactation consultant in the inpatient setting. Her research interests are early breastfeeding. She cofounded La Leche League (LLL) of Singapore and is a current LLL Leader in Idaho. She has been working with breastfeeding families since 1979.

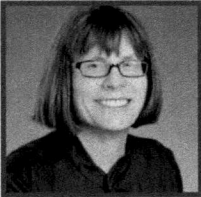

Jane Grassley, PhD, RN, IBCLC, is a professor in the School of Nursing, Boise State University and holds a joint appointment to assist nurses in the Saint Luke's Health System to conduct research related to breastfeeding support. She has been supporting breastfeeding for 40 years as a mother/baby nurse, and IBCLC the last 18 years.

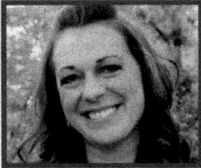

Kristen Koprowski, BSN, RN, is a recent graduate nurse from Boise State University where she focused her studies on breastfeeding support. She works as a family practice nurse as she pursues becoming an IBCLC.

USLCA

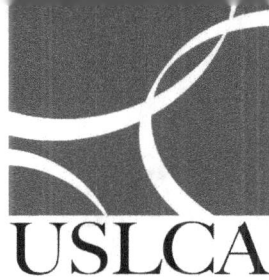

What Breastfeeding Mothers Want
Specific Contextualized Help

Amy Sarah Miller, BS | Anna Clarissa Jeanne Telford, BS
Brechtje Huizinga, BS | Manu Pinkster, BS
Jorieke ten Heggeler, BS | Joyce Elaine Miller, BS, DC, PhD

Keywords: breastfeeding, qualitative, maternal perceptions

Difficulty with breastfeeding in the newborn and new mother population is all too common, and too little is known about the type of healthcare assistance most relevant to these families. Therefore, 18 mothers were interviewed for their experiences with suboptimal breastfeeding and their perceptions of the healthcare they had received for the problem. These mothers attended an interdisciplinary breastfeeding clinic (midwifery and chiropractic) on the south coast of England. The goal of this study was to better understand mothers' preferences in healthcare resources to facilitate the most efficient and effective assistance to improve breastfeeding for mothers and infants. The main themes were that mothers desired ongoing reassurance and contextualized, nonconflicting advice that was specific to their baby.

Inability to breastfeed a newborn is a common and frustrating problem for families and their assisting healthcare professionals. The risks of not breastfeeding are legion and include the following:

- » Asthma
- » Atopic dermatitis
- » Celiac disease
- » Diabetes
- » Gastroenteritis
- » Inflammatory bowel disease
- » Lower respiratory tract infection
- » Necrotizing enterocolitis
- » Obesity
- » Otitis media
- » Respiratory syncytial virus—bronchiolitis
- » Sudden infant death syndrome (SIDS)
- » Upper respiratory tract infection (American Academy of Pediatrics, 2012)

The World Health Organization (WHO) guidelines recommend exclusive breastfeeding until 6 months of age (with breast milk continued alongside solid foods from that age onward) for the optimal lifelong health of both the child and mother (World Health Organization [WHO], 2013). Maternal benefits of breastfeeding include the following:

- » Decreased postpartum blood loss
- » Decreased postpartum depression
- » Decreased rate of child abuse
- » Decreased rate of breast cancer
- » Decreased rate of ovarian cancer
- » Decreased rate of uterine cancer
- » Increased child spacing with lactation amenorrhea
- » Rapid contraction of uterus after delivery (American Academy of Pediatrics, 2012)

In the United Kingdom, 84% of mothers initiate breastfeeding as soon after birth as possible (McAndrew et al., 2012). However, the rate of decline is precipitous: 69% at 1 week, 55% at 6 weeks, and 34% at 6 months of age for any breastfeeding. In terms of exclusive breastfeeding, the rates are even lower with 17% at 12 weeks and 12% continuing to 4 months of age (McAndrew et al., 2012).

One of the key reasons that mothers give for stopping is that they did not have sufficient help and support from the healthcare community to facilitate successful breastfeeding. National statistics shows that 80% of mothers who stop breastfeeding would have preferred to continue (McAndrew et al., 2012).

Costs of stopping breastfeeding are high in terms of the health of mother and baby as well as actual healthcare costs (Pokhrel et al., 2014). Their UK study estimated £11 million (US$16 million) annual savings in just four childhood infections (lower respiratory and gastrointestinal infections, otitis media, and necrotizing enterocolitis) if mothers were supported to breastfeed for 4 months. An estimated £31 million (US$46 million) could be saved in costs of maternal breast cancer by doubling the proportion of mothers breastfeeding for 7–18 months (Pokhrel et al., 2014). Studies from the United States have likewise determined that suboptimal breastfeeding may increase U.S. maternal morbidity and pediatric healthcare costs significantly (Bartick & Reinhold, 2010; Bartick et al., 2013). An estimated minimum of US$3.6 billion (in 1999 US$) would be saved if breastfeeding were increased to 50% at 6 months, by reducing the healthcare cost of treating only three conditions: otitis media, gastroenteritis, and necrotizing enterocolitis in the United States. This figure could be considerably higher if other conditions or maternal health issues related to breastfeeding were accounted for (Weimer, 2001). For a myriad of reasons, breastfeeding is best feeding, and all healthcare professionals must be vigilant to provide assistance.

The purpose of this study was to investigate what mothers say about care received and care needed for feeding difficulties, including their general perceptions about their experiences with healthcare professionals.

Method

This study evolved out of a larger study designed to create and validate an outcomes survey for parents accessing healthcare for their infants. Because a significant proportion of mothers interviewed had attended a breastfeeding clinic, it was important to document their specific needs and desires relative to the care accessed for the particular problem of breastfeeding. The purposes of this research were to identify the goals of the mother, the ways that healthcare professionals responded or did not respond to their needs, and to discover any themes that may lead to improved care for such mothers in the future.

This was designed as a qualitative study. Ethical approval was granted from an independent college ethics committee prior to the commencement of interviews. During August and September of 2014, mothers of infants attending an interdisciplinary breastfeeding clinic were interviewed. There was no specific recruitment other than to ask mothers at the end of their session if they would be willing to participate. Mothers could decline to participate. Informed consent was gained prior to interviews, which were semistructured, recorded anonymously, and completely confidential. Mothers were allowed to speak freely, and interviews lasted 10–30 minutes. Interview topics were the following:

» Impact of problem on mother and family
» Outcomes that the mother would like from care
» Time with healthcare professionals: What is her experience?

» Perceptions of the infant's problems

» Review of advice given: Is it useful?

» Experience of this exposure to the current feeding clinic

Interviews were transcribed verbatim and then analyzed by a team of six researchers, with a minimum of three members at a time. Content analysis was used for both quantitative and qualitative data collection (Wilkinson, 2011). Quantitative analysis was achieved by coding answers to each question and inputting the data from all participants to a spreadsheet. The qualitative analysis involved each team member individually deciding on the main themes of each transcript. The team then met, discussed, and agreed on final themes for each transcript. Categories were created (Ritchie, Spencer, & O'Connor, 2003) based on areas of healthcare that were apparent in the identified themes. Quotes that best represented each category were identified.

The setting was an outpatient, interdisciplinary midwifery and chiropractic breastfeeding clinic affiliated with a chiropractic teaching clinic and a British university on the south coast of England. Midwives and chiropractors are just two of many professions providing assistance with breastfeeding, each with their own areas of expertise. This clinic combines these two complementary approaches, aiming to provide their best possible assistance for the problem of suboptimal breastfeeding.

Results

Eighteen mothers agreed to participate. No mother refused to answer any of the questions. All mothers had presented for the problem of suboptimal breastfeeding for their baby. The characteristics of the mothers and babies were the following:

» Reason for presentation: suboptimal feeding

» Number previous professionals seen for the problem: mean: 7.7 (range: 2–17)

» Age of infants: 7–91 days; 14, younger than one month; 4, older than one month
» 16/18 mothers were primiparous
» 5/18 reported multiple interventions during birth
» 5/18 babies had tongue ties
» 12 female babies, 6 males
» 13 exclusively breastfed, 3 combination breast and formula milk, 2 exclusively formula fed

Mothers commented about the importance of breastfeeding and the difficulties of bottle feeding:

Yeah, I know the benefits of breastfeeding … not to mention it's easier to breastfeed, so that's why you know [I want] to breastfeed him.

I think it's the inability to provide and then the kind of for me it was having to formula feed, which was something I never wanted to do because I'm such a fan of breastfeeding, so it kind of had the guilt association with that and then it's the physical strain of feeding bottles, washing bottles, sterilizing bottles, expressing milk every 3 hours, it's just a nightmare, exhausting …

I can try and sleep when he sleeps during the day, but yeah, I don't know I think if I could feed him from the breast rather than expressing and doing bottles, which is a nightmare, then it'll be easier.

Yeah, it's the fact that I can't (breastfeed), I'm spending every 3 hours, I'm spending 45 minutes pumping, which I can't do whilst he's having a bottle on me, so I have to give him food and then get him to go to sleep, which will take about an hour and then pump for 40 minutes and then he'll be awake, like, in an hour, and then that's it, like, constantly, and that's a lot of stress.

Over the weekend, we stopped breastfeeding and went to bottles, it was just horrendous. We had lots of tears from everybody, big disruption . . . we couldn't leave the house.

The issue that I've got at the moment is . . . the time it takes me to get the bottle ready for her. Because very often I'm leaving her in the cot crying while I'm getting her feed ready, which is one of the reasons why I sort of, you know, ideally would like to breastfeed.

The mothers' comments about their experiences in this feeding clinic were generally positive, with emphasis on individualized help in a teamwork setting:

It was really reassuring and that is a vital thing.

I found here it's probably the most unhurried . . . and also a place where you get the advice just to you, not sat among a big group of people . . . so it did really help.

I'm quite a practical person, so I want to know kind of, like, specifics so it's like right, I've got a problem, what's the kind of resolution, what do I actually just need to do to make it work. And I think that that's been really helpful today.

I liked everyone was very friendly, welcoming, they explained what they were doing, why they were doing it, there's no pressure . . . and really helpful advice and supportive but not patronizing, which is a balance to get right.

In relation to this clinic . . . it's great, I think the two professions there to look at things from each individual point of view but work together.

It was very honest, it was really friendly. The professionals that I met were absolutely lovely, very honest, and very kind of open with everything and you could tell that they really wanted to be there.

It's just nice to be surrounded by people who know what they're doing.

I learned a lot from her (chiropractor) the first time we came last week about her feeding; you know just things that we wouldn't have known about if we'd not come here . . . No one would tell us that anywhere else, so it's quite nice to understand why she's doing the things she's doing now.

Everyone was listening, and when I asked the questions, I got answers and everything was explained.

Themes were broadly categorized under the mothers' report of likes and dislikes in healthcare and whether these were experienced or not. There were two main themes under their likes: reassurance and specific advice; there were two main themes classified as dislikes: stressors (with two categories: personal stressors and family stressors) and unsatisfactory healthcare resources (with three categories: poor continuity of care, insufficient time, and rules and pressures). Main themes are identified in bold, categories in italics, and quotes are indented. A subtheme of conflicting advice emerged in many interviews and was widely discussed as a stressful and difficult to manage entity. Conflicting advice was reported within and between professions, as well as from family and friends.

What Were Their Likes?

Reassurance

It's really important to be encouraged . . . to keep you going when you are having a bad day and you are thinking, "Oh God, I cannot do this anymore."

Reassurance is good because I think when you have kind of got worked up about it, or sort of worried that he wasn't eating . . . the reassurance is helpful that you are getting it and getting somewhere.

Specific Advice

I can look up generic advice on Google . . . I want somebody to actually look at her (the baby) and look at what we're doing and see if there's anything specific to us that can help.

Actually, what we need is somebody to sit down and watch us and correct us.

I want to know kind of like specifics, so it's like, right, I've got this problem, what's the kind of resolution, what can I actually do? I actually just need to make it work.

What Were Their Dislikes?

Stressors

The key elements of their personal stress were self-esteem issues around not being able to feed their baby, not knowing what to do with the baby around feeding, sleeping, and crying. Family stressors included isolation and trying to protect the rest of the family.

Personal Stress

They don't come with a manual!

I think it's (the great stress) the inability to provide.

The reality is so much less sleep. I thought if a baby feeds every 3 hours, then that meant that when you finished feeding, you had 3 hours, but I didn't realize that it took an hour to feed her, and then she doesn't sleep for more than an hour at a time.

I think it is the fact that he is completely inconsolable, so it doesn't actually matter what you do and again . . . it's not knowing and then having to accept that.

Family Stress

During the day, when I am dealing with it myself, I can kind of just get through it, but it's at night time that is the hardest because it is disturbing the sleep of my husband and that's not so great. So it's trying to make sure that he is happy . . . and that my husband is able to sleep . . . if it becomes frustrating, that's when we feel the most kind of change in our tension levels.

My husband had to go back to work, so I sent him off to the spare room because he has to get up at 5.

It's difficult, because the time she cries is the time my husband is at home.

Unsatisfactory Healthcare Resources

Poor Continuity of Care or Poor Care

I couldn't even say who my midwife is, I had so many. I haven't seen anyone twice, so I have never really established a relationship.

Tongue-tie: I've asked 3 people to look for it and all of them missed it, so it was only really my perseverance that meant that anyone saw it.

Insufficient Time

When they are halfway through a feed, you don't want somebody saying, "right, we need to let somebody else in now."

I was more conscious that I was taking up their time.

You go to a normal GP and you are rushed in 10 minutes, which obviously is never long enough, especially when you are new parents. We went in yesterday and we had about six or seven questions but . . . we felt we weren't getting much out of it.

Rules and Pressures

It's the very strict rules [for healthcare] . . . as a first time mom, I think too much of that, not letting you enjoy your baby.

I would like to enjoy it rather than feeling the pressure of weight gain.

The subtheme of conflicting advice was discussed in most interviews in response to various questions about multiple aspects of healthcare. Mothers generally found conflicting advice stressful and difficult to manage and viewed it as a negative outcome when seeking care.

In hospital, I had a lot of conflicting advice, which was quite frustrating . . . There would be a different midwife on duty who would come up with a completely different way of doing it.

I have been given different advice, which has been quite confusing . . . and I think . . . hindered at times, her feeding.

One of the most frustrating things is that everyone tells you something different, so that you don't know who's the one to believe.

Discussion

This study explores current perceptions and preferences of mothers of infants suffering from suboptimal breastfeeding. Most mothers wanted contextualized, specific advice, support, and help for their child. Mothers found general advice and competing advice stressful and, at times, felt it even hindered their progress. It is likely that this group of mothers is a special population, where general advice was insufficient to solve their feeding problems. This was demonstrated in the high average number (eight) of professionals consulted prior to entering this specialty clinic, which is most often accessed by direct referrals from other healthcare professionals (midwives, health visitors, tongue-tie clinic), who have presumably already given their assistance.

The mothers' main goals varied depending on their babies' age and the severity and chronicity of their problem. Mothers of babies with small problems usually wanted to fully resolve those issues. However, mothers of babies who had more severe or long-lasting feeding problems tended to be looking for an explanation as much as a resolution, and had perhaps accepted that they may not be able to continue breastfeeding exclusively. All planned to include breast milk in the baby's diet as long as physically and emotionally possible.

No matter what the problem, mothers wanted advice that was specific to their baby and found generic advice to be pedantic and self-serving, even "talking down" to the mother as though she hadn't tried to find her own answers. Their main desires were specific, individual advice for themselves and their babies and reassurance; they also wanted homework to help themselves and a brief, written record of the explanations received to remember and pass on information to family members. One of the main complaints mothers have about healthcare was the perceived lack of time, which restricted time to ask questions and to obtain full explanations. The mothers also disliked the lack of consistency in their care. They wished to see the same healthcare professional over time to allow an ongoing and trusting relationship to develop and to avoid conflicting advice, which was an ever-present irritation.

Mother's frustrations included general expectations that they could handle all aspects of caring for a new baby, even the second time around, although they did not feel fully equipped to do so ("they don't come with a manual"). They were protective of the rest of the family, particularly the father; the mothers bore the brunt of not only the feeding, which is logical, but also the excessive crying and sleep deprivation. When help arrived, reassurance was valued, except when it was not contextualized or sufficiently specific to answer their needs. Over and over, mothers did not value generic advice for feeding but wanted individual analysis of their problem. It seems that professionals, such as lactation consultants, with their high-level training, might be in the best position to offer this specificity. Yet most mothers in this cohort had not been able to access that level of help.

Conclusion

Mothers value support during breastfeeding in the forms of reassurance, specific individualized advice, and adequate time with a healthcare professional. Implementation of these areas of support may aid continuation of breastfeeding, benefiting the long-term health of both mother and infant.

References

American Academy of Pediatrics. (2012). Breastfeeding and the use of human milk. *Pediatrics, 129*(3), e827–e841. http://dx.doi .org/10.1542/ peds.2011-3552

Bartick, M., & Reinhold, A. (2010). The burden of suboptimal breastfeeding in the United States: A pediatric cost analysis. *Pediatrics, 125*(5), e1048–e1056. http://dx.doi.org/10.1542/ peds.2009-1616

Bartick, M. C., Stuebe, A. M., Schwarz, E. B., Luongo, C., Reinhold, A. G., & Foster, E. M. (2013). Cost analysis of maternal disease associated with suboptimal breastfeeding. *Obstetrics and Gynecology, 122*(1), 111–119.

McAndrew, F., Thompson, J., Fellows, L., Large, A., Speed, S., & Renfrew, M. J. (2012). *Infant feeding survey 2010.* Leeds, United Kingdom: Health and Social Care Information Centre.

Pokhrel, S., Quigley, M. A., Fox-Rushby, J., McCormick, F., Williams, A., Trueman, P., . . . Renfrew, M. J. (2015). Potential economic impacts from improving breastfeeding rates in the UK. *Archives of Disease in Childhood, 100*(4), 334–340. http://dx.doi.org/10.1136/archdischild-2014-306701

Ritchie, J., Spencer, S., & O'Connor, W. (2003). Carrying out qualitative research. In J. Ritchie & J. Lewis (Eds.), Qualitative research practice: A guide for social science students and researchers (pp. 219–262). London, United Kingdom: Sage. Weimer, D. (2001). The economic benefits of breastfeeding: A review and analysis. Retrieved from http://www.ers.usda.gov/publications/fanrr-food-assistance-nutrition-research-program/fanrr13.aspx#.UUoSezmGo1c

Wilkinson, S. (2011). Analyzing focus group data. In D. Silverman (Ed.), *Qualitative research: Issues of theory, method and practice* (3rd ed., pp. 168–184). London, United Kingdom: Sage.

World Health Organization. (2013). *Up to what age can a baby stay well nourished by just being breastfed?* Retrieved from http://www .who.int/features/qa/21/en/

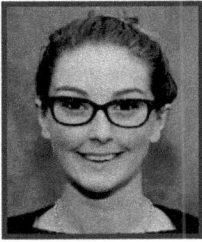

Amy Miller, BSc, is a chiropractic master's student with a special interest in the pediatric patient, particularly infant feeding and nutrition, and developmental delay. She is the lead of an interdisciplinary breast-feeding clinic at the Anglo-European College of Chiropractic, a student led initiative where midwives and chiropractors collaborate to provide support and care for the breastfeeding dyad.

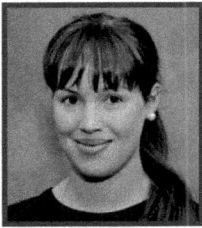

Anna Telford, BSc, is a 4th year master's student at the Anglo-European College of Chiropractic. She is passionate about providing chiropractic care to patients of all ages and backgrounds. She believes awareness should be raised among the public about the benefits of chiropractic care, from the pediatric patient through to the geriatric population.

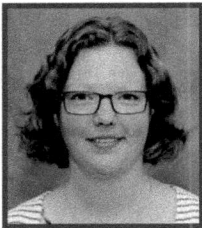

Brechtje Huizinga, BSc, is a 4th year master's student at the Anglo-European College of Chiropractic. She became interested in pediatrics after she saw what a difference it can make in someone's life. She believes breastfeeding is a key element for a healthy life and wants to promote this where she can. She is planning to set up breastfeeding sessions once she is out in practice.

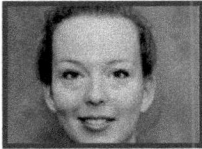

Manu Pinkster, BSc, originally from Holland, is currently a 4th year student at the Anglo-European College of Chiropractic. Her degree is in Human Sciences, and she is currently completing her Master's in Chiropractic.

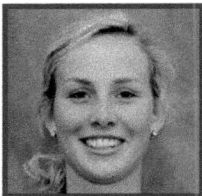

Jorieke ten Heggeler, BSc, is a 4th year master's student at the Anglo-European College of Chiropractic. She is passionate about providing care to patients who are in need, with a focus on pediatric patients and pregnant women. She believes that awareness should be raised among mothers about the huge benefits of breastfeeding. For the foreseeable future, she wants to promote greater education for mothers to empower them to make the best choices for their children's health.

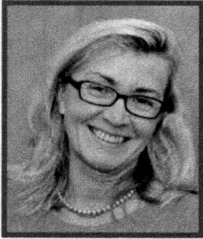

Joyce Miller, BSc, DC, PhD, is a pediatrics lecturer with more than 25 years practice experience. Currently an associate professor at Anglo-European College of Chiropractic in England, she oversees the busy feeding clinic in the teaching clinic and leads the University of Bournemouth's Master's Degree in Musculoskeletal Health-Pediatrics. Her PhD is in musculoskeletal health of the excessively crying baby. She is a certified Brazelton neonate examiner, and a diplomat of the RCPCH Nutrition Program.

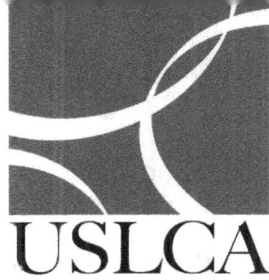

Where Are We Going Wrong?

Exploring and Identifying the Challenges to Exclusive Breastfeeding in a Tertiary-Care Facility

Sharanjit Kaur, MPH | Julie Smith-Fehr, RN, BScN, MN

Jana Stockham, RN, IBCLC | Angela Bowen, RN, PhD

Keywords: breastfeeding; lactation; human milk; milk banks; bottle-feeding; behavior

Despite efforts to achieve World Health Organization's best practice standards for a Baby-Friendly status, only 54% of babies discharged from a tertiary-care hospital in 2015 were exclusively breastfed. This is despite an initiation rate for breastfeeding of 92%. This report describes maternal and nurse beliefs about exclusive breastfeeding, supplementation, and human milk banking. To help us understand our high levels of formula supplementation, we surveyed 94 mothers and 75 nurses and found differing beliefs about formula supplementation and the use of human donor milk. Skin-to-skin and other policies were not being followed. Maternal and nurse breastfeeding education, along with up to date breastfeeding policies, are essential for organizations to meet the World Health Organization's standards to achieve Baby-Friendly status.

The World Health Organization (WHO) recommends exclusive breastfeeding for all infants for the first 6 months of life (WHO, 2003); however, exclusive breastfeeding rates often lag behind this goal (Health Canada, 2012). In 1992, the WHO and United Nations Children's Fund (UNICEF) launched the Baby-Friendly Hospital Initiative (BFHI), which outlines the Ten Steps to Successful Breastfeeding to protect, promote, and support breastfeeding (WHO, 2013). These ten steps include sustained improvement in institutional practices, training healthcare staff to implement policies, educate pregnant women about the benefits of breastfeeding, practice rooming-in, including skin-to-skin contact after birth, and avoid unnecessary formula supplementation (WHO, 2013).

Exclusive breastfeeding promotes the health and well-being of both mother and infant. It protects the baby from death and disease and provides physical, cognitive, and social support to the baby and its family (Health Canada, 2015). Exclusive breastfeeding includes human milk (expressed or donor), oral rehydration solution (ORS), and syrups (i.e., vitamins, minerals, and medicines), but it does not include supplementation with other feeding products (WHO, 2015).

Breastfeeding initiation rates vary internationally. In the United States, 81.1% of women initiate breastfeeding (Centers for Disease Control and Prevention, 2016); 70.1% in France (Organisation for Economic Co-operation and Development [OECD], 2009); 73.9% in England, (NHS England, 2013 to 2014); 97% in Norway (Australian Government Department of Health, 2012), and 96% in Australia (Australian Institute of Health and Welfare, 2011). In Canada, the breastfeeding initiation rate is 89% (Gionet, 2013); however, rates of exclusive breastfeeding at discharge are only 54% (Saskatoon Health Region [SHR], 2015) and are well below the WHO's recommended levels of 75% (WHO, 2014).

In our facility, 92% of women initiate breastfeeding within an hour after birth, but by discharge, the breastfeeding rate falls to 88% (SHR, 2015), and of this 88%, only 54% of babies were exclusively breastfed with 46% having been supplemented with formula (SHR, 2015). At the same time, infant formula use on the maternal–infant units increased from 13,022 bottles in 2013 to 21,254 in 2015 (SHR, 2015). The Human Milk Banking Association of North America (HMBANA) recommends that if the supply of maternal milk is insufficient, especially for the high-risk and premature infants, pasteurized human milk is the most appropriate supplementation. Milk banks play an important role in meeting needs of these babies (HMBANA, 2016). However, we do not have a formal supply of human donor milk for breast milk supplementation. As a result, in our community, human milk may be obtained from relatives, friends, or by human milk sharing on social media.

Hospital administrators sought to understand the reasons for the gap between the goals of the promoted BFHI policy and the infant feeding outcomes on the maternal–infant units in our region that includes a tertiary-care hospital and home visiting community program: specifically, the low rates of exclusive breastfeeding and high rates of supplementation. Therefore, we explored maternal and nurse knowledge and beliefs about exclusive breastfeeding, the reasons for supplementation, and the use of a human milk bank.

Method

This cross-sectional study involved mothers and nurses from maternal–infant units within a tertiary-care Canadian hospital and home visiting community program with more than 5,500 live births in 2015.

Participants

Participants included a convenience sample of nurses from our maternal–infant units and mothers from the in-patient post-partum ward maternal–infant units. Approval was received from the BLINDED Health Region and BLINDED University Behavioral Ethics Committees. Informed consent was received from all participants.

Inclusion and Exclusion Criteria

Women 18 years or older, who speak English, or had a family member available to translate the survey were included. The goal of the study was to identify the challenges to exclusive breastfeeding. Therefore, we only included mothers whose babies had received formula supplementation during their in-patient stay. Exclusively breastfeeding mothers whose infants had not received supplementation were excluded from the study. All nurses who worked on the maternal–infant units were invited to participate with no exclusions.

Data Collection

Mothers were interviewed and filled out the questionnaires in their in-patient room prior to discharge home, over a 2-week period. Nurses were asked to complete the survey during their work shifts. Data were also gathered from the maternal and infant in-patient charts.

Questionnaire

The mother's interview included 22 questions, including age, gravida, gestational age, and weight of the baby at birth. We asked about challenges the mothers faced to exclusively breastfeed, the reasons for supplementation, and views about human milk as an alternative source of nutrition for their baby. The nurses' survey tested their breastfeeding knowledge via 20 multiple-choice questions. We also asked their beliefs on exclusive breastfeeding, formula supplementation, free formula supply to hospital, and the use of human milk banking.

Analysis

Descriptive statistics were used. The nurses' knowledge was divided into three categories: those below 50%, those between 51% and 75%, and those who scored up to 100%. Data were analyzed using the latest version of SPSS.

Results

Mothers

Ninety-four mothers were interviewed; 67% (*n*=63) of women had vaginal deliveries, and 14% (*n*=14) of those were vacuum assistance. Fifty-seven percent (*n*=54) of the women were primigravidas, 40% of mothers (*n*=38) were multigravidas, and 3% (*n*=2) of women did not answer this question (Table 1). Seventy-four percent (*n*=70) of the mothers stated their babies received supplementation because of a medical condition. Eleven percent (*n*=10) stated that supplementing their baby was personal choice, and 13% (*n*=12) of the women did not know why their babies had received formula. Forty-five percent (*n*=42) of the mothers stated inadequate milk supply was their biggest breastfeeding challenge, followed by breast pain 14% (*n*=14), sore nipples 11% (*n*=11), and infant tongue-tie 11% (*n*=10).

Of the multiparous mothers, 63% (*n*=24) had also supplemented their first baby. Fifteen percent (*n*=15) of mothers practiced skin-to-skin contact after delivery, whereas 40% (*n*=37) were separated from their babies, but this was for less than 20 minutes,

10% (*n*=9) of mothers did not have any skin-to-skin contact with their babies despite not being separated from them after birth. The in-patient charts showed that the main reason noted for supplementation was low blood sugar at 36% (*n*=33), followed by admission to neonatal care 32% (*n*=30). Factors such as maternal illness and infant dehydration were minor, contributing 4.2% (*n*=4) and 6.3% (*n*=6), respectively.

Almost half (*n*=48) of the mothers stated that pasteurized human milk from a milk bank would be the preferred method to supplement their baby. Half of mothers (50%) were unsure about using human milk from a milk bank because of the unknown medical history of the donor mother and lack of knowledge regarding pasteurization of the collected milk. Two mothers reported using unpasteurized donor human milk for their baby, and 3 were using home methods of pasteurized human milk. The remaining 84 denied accessing any human milk for supplementation.

Nurses

Seventy-five nurses completed the survey; 95% (*n*=72) answered more than 50% of the multiple-choice questions correctly, that is, 45% (*n*=34) scored up to 100% and 50% (*n*=38) scored up to 75%, only 5% (*n*=3) of the nurses received a mark less than 50%. Fifty-two percent (*n*=39) of the nurses reported that they do not have enough time to teach mothers about exclusive breastfeeding, 42% (*n*=32) said they sometimes have time, whereas only 5% agreed that they do get enough time to educate mothers about exclusive breastfeeding. Most nurses stated that infant formula use was mostly because of mother's choice (62%, *n*=47), followed by medical reasons (37%, *n*=28), inadequate education to mothers (25%, *n*=19), and the availability of free infant formula (6%, *n*=5).

Table 1. Demographic Findings	% (n)
Age (years)	
18–24	26.60 (25)
25–34	50.00 (47)
35–44	20.21 (19)
45 or older	2.13 (2)
Type of delivery	
Spontaneous vaginal	52.13 (49)
Caesarean	31.91 (30)
Vacuum assisted	14.89 (14)
Gestational age of baby	
Less than 32 weeks	2.13 (2)
Less than 37 weeks	30.85 (29)
37 weeks or after	65.96 (62)
Weight of baby at the time of birth	
<1,500 g	3.19 (3)
1,500 g to <2,500 g	27.66 (26)
>2,500 g	67.02 (63)
Is this your first baby?	
Yes	57.40 (54)
No	40.40 (38)
No answer	3.00 (2)
If this is not your first baby, was one of your other babies supplemented?	
Yes	63.20 (24)
No	36.80 (14)
Why was your baby supplemented with formula?	
Medical reasons	74.47 (70)
Personal choice	10.64 (10)
Fussy baby	8.51 (8)
I don't know	12.77 (12)

Almost two-thirds (n=47) of the nurses said that breastfeeding is better for babies than infant formula, whereas 29% (n=22) stated that formula is a very good alternative to breast milk. Eight percent of nurses (n=6) think that maternal preference should be the only deciding factor for formula use. Last, 90% (n=70) of nurses stated that a human milk bank would be beneficial for both mothers and infants.

Mother–Nurse Comparison

There were notable differences between the mothers' and nurses' knowledge and beliefs; 62% (n=47) of nurses think that for the majority of babies, infant formula is given as a result of the mother's personal choice. Of the mothers interviewed, only 11% (n=10) stated it was their personal choice. Only 37% of the nurses said that infant formula use was because of a medical condition of the mother or baby. However, 74% (n=70) of the mothers interviewed believed the baby was supplemented because of medical condition. These examples show a discrepancy in beliefs. When asked about use of a human milk bank for supplementation, 90% of nurses said it would be a good strategy, whereas only 50% of the mothers interviewed responded positively about using a human milk bank.

Discussion

Our study supports the findings of DiGirolamo, Grummer-Strawn, and Fein (2003) who state that mothers have a perceived rather than actual inadequate milk supply. In addition, nurses' lack of knowledge about breastfeeding contributes to poor patient education about breastfeeding. This in addition to the free formula supplied to the hospital all contribute to low rates of exclusive breastfeeding.

Lack of breastfeeding knowledge is an ongoing concern for new mothers. The perception of insufficient milk production was a major concern voiced by the mothers in our study. This affirms Gatti (2008) who reports that the perception of lack of milk production is a leading issue for women across Canada.

According to UNICEF, the introduction of infant formula early in a baby's life reduces the chances a mother will resume exclusive breastfeeding (UNICEF, 2015). A 2015 study found that when hospitals had a policy of not accepting free infant formula, in-hospital formula supplementation was reduced and exclusive breastfeeding rates increased (Tarrant et al., 2015). At the time of this study, this tertiary-care hospital is accepting free formula. Therefore, it is essential for administrators to realize that following the International Code of Marketing of Breast-Milk Substitutes for supplementation discourages the increasing use of formula (WHO, 2003), which might be contributing to the current low rates of exclusive breastfeeding.

The literature suggests that immediate, uninterrupted skin-to-skin contact for a minimum of an hour is one of the most effective interventions to promote exclusive breastfeeding and to elevate infant blood sugar levels (Crenshaw, 2014). This supports our findings that 10% of the babies in our study did not remain in skin-to-skin contact despite no obvious cause for being separated from their mother (i.e., for maternal or infant medical reasons) and that most babies who were supplemented was because of low blood sugar level.

Repeating information to mothers and nurses about exclusive breastfeeding, milk expression, and proper supplementation (including access to human milk) can increase exclusive breastfeeding rates to the WHO standards of 75% exclusive breastfeeding and make achieving Baby-Friendly status possible (Martens, 2000). Our study also suggests that when women do not fully understand when or how to supplement, it likely impacts the rates of exclusive breastfeeding. This appears to have been influenced by the nurses who stated that they do not have time to teach the mothers about exclusive breastfeeding. Prenatal classes are an ideal venue to teach women about the importance of breastfeeding, options for supplementation, and to influence their beliefs about exclusive breastfeeding (Centers for Disease Control and Prevention, 2013).

Limitations

The mothers may have been concerned that their answers may reflect poorly on their mothering abilities and answered accordingly, which may have contributed to social desirability bias. Second, the small sample size may affect the generalizability of results, although the sample was consistent with the usual population of the unit. Third, a few mothers were not fluent in English, so family members gave answers on their behalf. Some might have understood the questions differently than was intended or did not want family to know their actual responses. Last, data were not divided by area of work; the maternal–infant in-patient area is staffed mostly with registered nurses, whereas the home visiting community program has predominantly registered nurses also trained as IBCLCs, with different knowledge, roles, and skill set.

Conclusion

This study provides insights into the challenges faced in trying to achieve exclusive breastfeeding and subsequent Baby-Friendly status in a tertiary-care facility. This includes gaps in the knowledge and beliefs of mothers and nurses related to exclusive breastfeeding and supplementation. Mothers need to understand the importance of exclusive breastfeeding and the practices that promote it, such as appropriate supplementation, skin-to-skin contact, and human milk banking. Nurses need appropriate orientation, continuing education, and annual updates on best practices in breastfeeding. And they need to take the time to ensure that postpartum mothers have the information necessary to make informed decisions about exclusive breastfeeding and avoid misperceptions about formula supplementation and human milk options.

Increasing maternal and nursing knowledge, supporting existing policy, access to human donor milk, and policy changes to not receive formula free are essential to improve exclusive breastfeeding rates in order to meet the WHO's standards to achieve Baby-Friendly status.

References

Australian Government Department of Health. (2012). *An international comparison study into the implementation of the WHO code and other breastfeeding initiatives.* Norway—the WHO code and breastfeeding: An international comparative overview. Retrieved from http://www.health.gov.au/internet/publications/publishing.nsf/Content/int-comp-whocode-bf-init~int-comp-whocode-bfinit-ico|int-comp-whocode-bf-init-ico-norway

Australian Institute of Health and Welfare. (2011). *2010 Australian National Infant Feeding Survey: Indicator results.* Canberra, Australian Capital Territory Australia: Author. Retrieved from http://www.aihw.gov.au/publicationdetail/?id=10737420927

Carroll, K. (2014). Body dirt or liquid gold? How the 'safety' of donated breastmilk is constructed for use in neonatal intensive care. *Social Studies of Science, 44*(3), 466–485. Retrieved from https://www.ncbi.nlm.nih.gov/pubmed/25051591

Centers for Disease Control and Prevention. (2013). *Strategies to prevent obesity and other chronic diseases: The CDC guide to strategies to support breastfeeding mothers and babies.* Atlanta, GA: U.S. Department of Health and Human Services. Retrieved from https://www.cdc.gov/breastfeeding/pdf/BF-Guide-508.PDF

Centers for Disease Control and Prevention. (2016). *Breastfeeding report card: Progressing toward national breastfeeding goals.* United

States, 2016. Retrieved from https://www.cdc.gov/breastfeeding/pdf/2016breastfeedingreportcard.pdf

Crenshaw, J. T. (2014). Healthy Birth Practice #6: Keep mother and baby together—it's best for mother, baby, and breastfeeding. *The Journal of Perinatal Education, 23*(4), 211–217. Retrieved from http://dx.doi.org/10.1891/1058-1243.23.4.211

DiGirolamo, A. M., Grummer-Strawn, L. M., & Fein, S. B. (2003). Do perceived attitudes of physicians and hospital staff affect breastfeeding decisions? *Birth, 30*(2), 94–100.

Gatti, L. (2008). Maternal perceptions of insufficient milk supply in breastfeeding. *Journal of Nursing Scholarship, 40*(4), 355–363. http://dx.doi.org/10.1111/j.1547-5069.2008.00234.x

Gionet, L. (2013). *Health at a glance. Breastfeeding trends in Canada.* Ottawa, Ontario, Canada: Statistics Canada. Retrieved from http://www.statcan.gc.ca/pub/82-624-x/2013001/article/ 11879-eng.htm

Health Canada. (2012). *Duration of exclusive breastfeeding in Canada: Key statistics and graphics (2009-2010).* Retrieved from http://www.hcsc.gc.ca/fnan/surveill/nutrition/commun/prenatal/exclusive-exclusif-eng.php#share

Health Canada. (2015). *Nutrition for healthy term infants: Recommendations from birth to six months.* Retrieved from http://www.hc-sc.gc.ca/fn-an/nutrition/infant-nourisson/ recom/index-eng.php Human Milk Banking Association of North America. (2016). Retrieved from https://www.hmbana.org/

Martens, P. J. (2000). Does breastfeeding education affect nursing staff beliefs, exclusive breastfeeding rates, and Baby-Friendly Hospital Initiative compliance? The experience of a small, rural Canadian hospital. *Journal of Human Lactation, 16*(4), 309–318. http://dx.doi.org/10.1177/089033440001600407

NHS England. (2014). Statistical release: Breastfeeding initiation & breastfeeding prevalence 6-8 weeks. *Revised Quarter 4 2013/14.* Retrieved from https://www.england.nhs.uk/statistics/wp-content/uploads/sites/2/2014/03/Breastfeeding-1314-Revised-Data.pdf

Organisation for Economic Co-operation and Development. (2009). *CO1.5: Breastfeeding rates.* Retrieved from https://www.oecd .org/els/family/43136964.pdf

Saskatoon Health Region. (2015). Baby-friendly initiative external assessment of CHS (Report no. 24A).

Tarrant, M., Lok, K., Fong, D., Lee, I., Sham, A., Lam, C., . . .
Dodgson, J. (2015). Effect of a hospital policy of not accepting free
infant formula on in-hospital formula supplementation rates and
breast-feeding duration. *Public Health Nutrition, 18*(14), 2689–2699.
http://dx.doi.org/10.1017/S1368980015000117

United Nations Children's Fund. (2015). Breastfeeding. Retrieved
from http://www.unicef.org/nutrition/index_24824.html

World Health Organization. (1981). *International code of marketing
of breast-milk substitutes. Retrieved* from http://www.who.int/
nutrition/publications/code_english.pdf

World Health Organization. (1998). *Evidence for the ten steps to
successful breastfeeding.* Geneva, Switzerland: Author.
Retrieved from http://www.who.int/nutrition/publications/
evidence_ten_step_eng.pdf

World Health Organization. (2014). Implementation of the
BabyFriendly Hospital Initiative. Retrieved from
http://www.who.int/ elena/bbc/implementation_bfhi/en/

World Health Organization. (2015). The World Health
Organization's infant feeding recommendation. Retrieved
from http://www.who .int/nutrition/topics/infantfeeding_
recommendation/en/

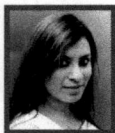

Sharanjit Kaur, MPH, is a public health professional with a master's degree from the University of Saskatchewan. She has a keen interest in addressing major health issues in aboriginal and vulnerable populations.

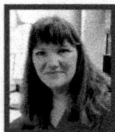

Julie Smith-Fehr, RN, BScN, MN, is a nurse manager with more than 30 years of nursing. Julie has a passion for ensuring that mothers and newborns receive best practice family centered care.

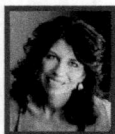

Jana Stockham, RN, IBCLC, has worked as a registered nurse for more than 20 years and as an IBCLC for 18 years. She has a passion to help families with new babies and has been trained as a Baby-Friendly assessor.

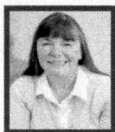

Angela Bowen, RN, PhD, is a professor of nursing with an extensive background practicing and teaching maternity care. Her research focuses on factors affecting maternal mental health and well-being.

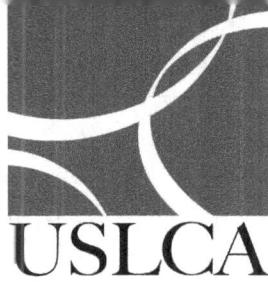

Improving Communication and Collaboration Between Lactation Consultants and Doctors for Better Breastfeeding Outcomes

A Review

Janice Fyfe, B. Comm (Hons), ND

Shelagh Quinn, IBCLC | Tristan Kiraly, RN, IBCLC

Edith Kernerman, IBCLC, RLC

Keywords: communication, lactation consultants, physicians, interprofessional relationships, barriers

The goal of this review is to evaluate the most effective methods of professional interaction, collaboration, and communication between lactation consultants and other healthcare professionals for optimal patient care. The literature revealed that for effective interprofessional communication, lactation consultants must communicate and promote a clear understanding of breastfeeding challenges, their solutions, how lactation consultants can help establish and maintain a positive breastfeeding experience for both mother and baby, preferred modes of communication, as well as the common terminology used by lactation consultants.

It is imperative that lactation consultants (International Board Certified Lactation Consultant [IBCLC]) are able to collaborate with other healthcare professionals to ensure that breast-feeding mothers and their infants get the highest quality of care and ensured safety. Effective communication methods, as well as the universal understanding of professional language between lactation consultants and other healthcare professionals, have yet to be determined. The goal of this research is to evaluate the most effective methods of interaction and use of breastfeeding-specific terms to optimize communication between lactation consultants and other healthcare professionals including, but not limited to, family physicians; pediatricians; ear, nose, and throat physicians; midwives; naturopathic doctors; and chiropractors. The research on this particular topic relating directly to lactation consultants and their interprofessional relationships is extremely limited. Thus, we had to broaden our search criteria to include all interprofessional collaboration. To assess the existing research that relates to this topic, studies and other journal articles relating to healthcare professionals' attitudes and beliefs about breast-feeding, as well as the benefits and barriers to interprofessional collaboration, were evaluated.

Physicians are the gatekeepers for the availability of many services for patients (Jabbar, 2011). It is often left up to them to decide what care their patient needs and who is best suited to provide that service to them. This system creates barriers because each healthcare profession possesses its own culture and values resulting in a lack of common understanding of issues and unfamiliarity with each other's vocabulary and problem-solving approaches (Hall, 2005). Professions have struggled to define their boundaries, identity, sphere of practice, and role in patient care. For example, the main outcome valued by physicians is to save a patient's life (Hall, 2005), not necessarily to improve quality of life. In order for interprofessional collaboration to work, physicians must value the type of work being done. If not, they will not be enthusiastic members of the team (Hall, 2005). It is important that professionals have an understanding of each other's scope of practice and expertise because interprofessional teamwork is becoming increasingly recognized and may result in improved job satisfaction (Hall, 2005).

Other barriers that restrict professional collaboration include external factors like the healthcare system and financial pressures. Many services are not covered and therefore create an out-of-pocket expense for patients. Power relationships are also a barrier, and simple uses of particular language such as "my patient" create a power imbalance that leads to a difficult work dynamic (Jabbar, 2011).

Gaboury, Bujold, Boon, and Moher (2009) interviewed 21 practitioners from Integrative Health Centres across Canada and found that collaboration is more likely to occur if there are similar interests and philosophies. Furthermore, they found that professional maturity and intellectual curiosity are paramount as personality traits in order for one to have the capacity to recognize one's own limits and give patients an appropriate referral for safer care (Gaboury et al., 2009). This study also recognized that additional barriers imposed by the licensing boards have very specific standards of care that may inhibit optimal patient care (Gaboury et al., 2009). It also found that a basic understanding and knowledge of other's fields of expertise is critical for team cohesion. One of the participants in the study stated,

> The more that each individual knows what type of things that we handle, what types of things we do, then it makes it easier for me to utilize someone else within the facility, when I am faced with that decision.

This understanding must also include common terminology within the various professions to be widely understood, whether they are sharing patient charts or letters back and forth. The ability to use common medical language must be a prerequisite to interprofessional collaboration as well as the willingness of the various professions to learn from each other (Gaboury et al., 2009). Although Gaboury et al. (2009) had a relatively small sample size and did not discuss the structure of collaboration within the various clinics, the findings are still relevant.

Interprofessional Communication

The importance of language was an overarching theme among many articles. A small survey of general physicians in England found that professional jargon can be a barrier to effective communication with chiropractors and osteopaths. Terms that can be misunderstood because of differences in interpretation are potentially even more damaging than a complete unfamiliarity with a term in general, illustrating that familiarity does not necessarily translate to understanding (Breen, Carrington, Collier, & Vogel, 2000). Another study looked at the comanaged care of palliative patients with physicians and nurses in three different settings: community, hospital, and hospice. They found that the nurse's ability to speak using medical terminology was key to a functional working relationship (Street & Blackford, 2001).

In a study aimed specifically at communication patterns between complementary and alternative medicine (CAM) and biomedical practitioners, they found that

> *individuals engage in knowledge sharing and creative problem solving only when they have already established a language in which they can combine and exchange their*

existing knowledge. (Soklaridis, Kelner, Love, & Cassidy, 2009)

The conclusion of the study found that the "commonality of understanding language should be the initial focus of improving communication between biomedical and CAM practitioners" (Soklaridis et al., 2009).

A referral letter from other healthcare professionals was the preferred form of communication by physicians (Schiff et al., 2011). Within these letters, providing evidence-based medicine with recommendations or justification for treatment plans increased healthcare professional's credibility with that particular physician. This further fosters a positive working relationship and familiarity with that health practitioner's profession and scope of practice (Schiff et al., 2011).

Schoop (1999) conducted a study that evaluated how to create information technology based on the language/action perspective and to support multidisciplinary written communication and cooperation in healthcare. The study was conducted using interviews with nurses and physicians. The results found that collaboration is important. Nurses and physicians have different roles, tasks, and professional interests. And there are communication problems (more so with written communication), different terminologies, and they communicate in different modes, including ward rounds and case conferences. They found that oral communication has more opportunity to rephrase, or increase understanding of terminology, whereas written communication leaves more room for lack of understanding and miscommunication between doctors and nurses (Schoop, 1999). This is less relevant for lactation consultants, who typically do not work alongside physicians in the same environment. The study found that a computer system could use linguistic programming to translate communication between the two professionals to make the language used with each other more understandable during written communication (Schoop, 1999).

Physicians' Breastfeeding Education, Knowledge, and Practices

Physician recommendations and confidence play a key role in breastfeeding care, yet there has been some disconnect between World Health Organization (WHO) recommendations and physician education to effectively support patients in achieving these standards (Schanler, O'Connor, & Lawrence, 1999).

To assess physician's current beliefs and breastfeeding values, Schanler et al. (1999) sampled 1,602 American Academy of Pediatrics fellows at random. They received a 71% response rate. Some of the breastfeeding recommendations identified were exclusive breastfeeding for the first month after birth (65%), breastfeeding for up to 1 year (37%), and routine recommendation of some form of supplementation (22%). Only 44% recommended that the infant be put to the breast within a half hour after delivery, 59% felt the infant should be fed on demand, 31% recommended feeding 8–12 times per day, and 23% advised against the use of pacifiers until breastfeeding was well established. Twenty-eight percent of respondents indicated that they would discontinue breastfeeding for breast and/or nipple problems, and 30% recommended semi-solid foods before 5 months of age. Most common reasons for not recommending breastfeeding included medical conditions, such as mastitis, nipple problems, low milk supply, jaundice, and low weight gain. These conditions have recognized therapeutic approaches that generally do not preclude breastfeeding. In addition, the majority agreed, or was neutral, in reference to the idea that breastfeeding and formula feeding are equivalent (Schanler et al., 1999).

Schanler et al. (1999) also found that education played a role in pediatrician's confidence in providing breastfeeding care. Fifty-eight percent of pediatricians had some education on breastfeeding management while in medical school or residency. These practitioners were more likely to be younger than 45 years of age and female. Respondents who attended any educational event that focused on breastfeeding management were significantly more confident in their abilities to manage common breastfeeding challenges; however, they were not found to necessarily be more knowledgeable about breastfeeding. More important, most respondents had not attended information sessions on breastfeeding management in the last 3 years and wanted more education on breastfeeding management (Schanler et al., 1999).

Sixty percent of respondents had children who were breastfed, and pediatricians with personal experience said they were more confident (87% said very confident) in their ability to manage common breastfeeding problems than pediatricians without personal experience (67%). The authors' findings and conclusion indicated that pediatricians have significant educational needs in the area of breastfeeding management (Schanler et al., 1999).

Health professionals who focus on the medical-risk perspective in the mother–infant dyad want more control of breastfeeding and may put less trust in the dyad's ability to manage breastfeeding (Ekström, Matthiesen, Widström, & Nissen, 2005). However, it was not studied if those professionals who have more confidence in managing breastfeeding may feel a sense of increased control and thus trust that the dyad can successfully manage breastfeeding (Ekström et al., 2005).

These results were further verified in the United States by a national and statewide survey study, published in Public

Health Reports, that showed how education to all staff members in 13 clinics, including administration staff, improved breastfeeding knowledge, attitudes, and practices (Khoury, Hinton, Mitra, Carothers, & Foretich, 2002). The researchers were able to achieve these results through implementation of a training program entitled, "How to Support a Breastfeeding Mother." The program was designed specifically to address the barriers that mothers experience with breastfeeding, and the type of support they need to overcome them, and the needs of breastfeeding support previously identified in mail-out surveys. The training was divided into three levels, including one 1.5-hour workshop and an additional two 3-hour workshops. These workshops discussed benefits and barriers to breastfeeding, breastfeeding counseling through the early days postpartum and during breastfeeding challenges, and special situations, including medical issues affecting the infant and/ or mother, with education on various devices and methods for storing human milk. The clinics with the intervention showed improvement in all primary outcome variables including knowledge, attitudes and beliefs, and confidence about breastfeeding versus the 13 clinics in the control group (Khoury et al., 2002).

The Professional Relationship Between Physicians and Lactation Consultants

Challenges experienced by the breastfeeding dyad can be addressed by referring to a lactation consultant. Research by Williams (1995) focused on increasing the credibility of lactation consultants in the eyes of physicians to foster positive interprofessional relationships and encourage referrals to best provide patient care. There were 10 variables found to be most critical for lactation consultants to effectively communicate with physicians: (a) identify oneself in person (if possible), identify extent of training, and offer in-house training; (b) relate information in a way the physician understands— concise, start with chief complaint, and include history of present condition, past history, family history, social history, physical findings, assessment, impression, and plan; (c) discuss the risk/benefit ratio of the plan for the dyad, and if the treatment is unconventional, or may be new to the doctor, briefly summarize any scientific evidence to support the treatments (or if evidence is limited, state personal clinical observations); (d) cite supporting studies from medical journals if possible, otherwise from well-designed studies, whatever the journal is; (e) provide the single most appropriate journal article where appropriate; (f) know what you want from the physician for each case—be specific about what action you recommend/ request and be concise, and have articles cited to back up the request; (g) show that you respect the physician's opinion/diagnosis and that you are on the same page; (h) follow up closely and maintain communication; (i) adapt to the personalities of the doctor (e.g., one may want detailed updates and another brief); and (j) increase credibility by making good judgments, maintaining close follow-up with the client, and maintaining good communication because these will increase the likelihood of future referrals from the same physician, as well as new referrals from colleagues.

As research by Williams (1995) previously noted, relating information in a way that a physician communicates is important, including units of measure. Most physicians use grams and kilograms to measure weight, so all correspondence with them should be consistent in communicating weights in these units to avoid confusion and additional conversion.

Conclusion

The current research on interprofessional relationships high-lights the importance of the views and beliefs held by various team members, particularly physicians, about other health-care professional's area of medicine. This often dictates their openness and enthusiasm to collaborate in patient care. It is critical that team members from various professions have an understanding and familiarity of the work each other does, education they hold, and the language one another uses to promote and encourage collaboration and referrals to one another. Preferred methods of communication between professionals, particularly physicians, seem to favor a written letter, unless those professionals are working side by side on a daily basis, then dialogue seemed to work best.

Mother and infant dyads are a patient population with specific needs that make them unique from all others. Views and beliefs about breastfeeding, as well as confidence in supporting breastfeeding mothers, improved among physicians and other healthcare providers, with more education and understanding about the needs and challenges of this patient population. Unfortunately, the research has also revealed that many healthcare providers have not been adequately exposed to this important education and training.

The WHO guidelines recommend breastfeeding because of its benefits over other feeding alternatives. It is clear that if physicians, as gatekeepers, support these recommendations in their professional practice, and therefore support mothers in the breastfeeding process, they must learn about the risks of not breastfeeding. If they don't have this education, breast-feeding challenges are not adequately identified, addressed, or managed, and the risks of not breastfeeding are too easily disregarded. Challenges experienced by the breastfeeding dyad can be addressed by referring to a lactation consultant, but in order for this important collaboration to be effective, there must be an understanding of the profession, educational requirements, and language used by lactation consultants.

It is clear from the literature reviewed that in order for lactation consultants to work alongside physicians in the care of patients to optimize breastfeeding, physicians must have a clear understanding of breastfeeding challenges, their solutions, how lactation consultants can help establish and maintain a positive breastfeeding experience for both mother and baby, preferred mode of communication, as well as the common terminology used by lactation consultants to establish an effective interprofessional relationship. This research has yet to be conducted, and the establishment of this professional relationship is imperative for optimal patient care.

References

Breen, A., Carrington, M., Collier, R., & Vogel, S. (2000). Communication between general and manipulative practitioners: A survey. *Complementary Therapies in Medicine, 8,* 8–14.

Ekström, A., Matthiesen, A. S., Widström, A. M., & Nissen, E. (2005). Breastfeeding attitudes among counselling health professionals: Development of an instrument to describe breastfeeding attitudes. *Scandinavian Journal of Public Health, 33,* 353–359.

Gaboury, I., Bujold, M., Boon, H., & Moher, D. (2009). Interprofessional collaboration within Canadian integrative healthcare clinics: Key components. *Social Science & Medicine, 69,* 707–715.

Hall, P. (2005). Interprofessional teamwork: Professional cultures as barriers. *Journal of Interprofessional Care, 19*(Suppl. 1), 188–196.

Jabbar, A. (2011). Language, power and implications for interprofessional collaboration: Reflections on a transition from social work to medicine. *Journal of Interprofessional Care, 25*(6), 447–448.

Khoury, A. J., Hinton, A., Mitra, A. K., Carothers, C., & Foretich, C. (2002). Improving breastfeeding knowledge, attitudes, and practices of WIC clinic staff. *Public Health Reports, 117,* 453–462.

Schanler, R., O'Connor, K., & Lawrence, R. (1999). Pediatricians' practices and attitudes regarding breastfeeding promotion. *Pediatrics, 103*(3), E35.

Schiff, E., Frenkel, M., Shilo, M., Levy, M., Schachter, L., Freifeld, Y., . . . Ben-Arye, E. (2011). Bridging the physician and CAM practitioner communication gap: Suggested framework for communication between physicians and CAM practitioners based on a cross professional survey from Israel. *Patient Education and Counseling, 85,* 188–193.

Schoop, M. (1999). An empirical study of multidisciplinary communication in healthcare using a language-action perspective. *The Language Action Perspective,* 59–72.

Soklaridis, S., Kelner, M., Love, R., & Cassidy, D. (2009). Integrative health care in a hospital setting: Communication patterns between CAM and biomedical practitioners. *Journal of Interprofessional Care, 23*(6), 655–667.

Street, A., & Blackford, J. (2001). Communication issues for the interdisciplinary community palliative care team. *Journal of Clinical Nursing, 10,* 643–650.

Williams, E. (1995). Increasing your credibility with physicians: Strategies for lactation consultants. *Journal of Human Lactation, 11*(1), 3–4

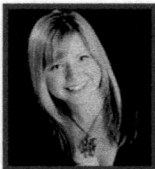

Janice Fyfe, B. Comm (Hons), ND, is a graduate of the Asper School of Business at the University of Manitoba and is a doctor of naturopathic medicine, having studied at the Canadian College of Naturopathic Medicine. She is also pursuing her designation as an IBCLC, having completed the lactation medicine program at the International Breastfeeding Centre.

Shelagh Quinn, IBCLC, studied lactation medicine at the International Breastfeeding Centre before completing her board exams. She is now a private practice clinician in Toronto.

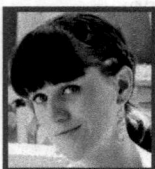

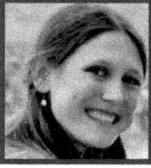

Tristan Kiraly, RN, IBCLC, is a Registered Nurse and completed the lactation medicine program at the International breastfeeding Centre before acquiring her IBCLC certification. She currently works in private practice in York region, Ontario.

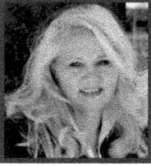

Edith Kernerman, IBCLC, RLC, is a clinician, educator, and researcher in the field of lactation medicine. Kernerman specializes in breast pain assessment and treatment, tethered oral tissue in babies, and inability to latch.

USLCA

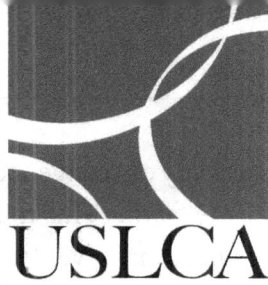

Using Avatars to Enhance Breastfeeding Education for Undergraduate Nursing Students

Jeanie Flood, PhD, RN, IBCLC

Kathleen Commendador, PhD, WHNP-BC

Keywords: avatar, nursing students, breastfeeding skills, nursing education

Maternal–child health courses must cover the perinatal period from preconception to postpartum. Nursing students must learn skills for labor support, as well as postpartum care, including the support and promotion of breastfeeding. Students have limited opportunities to practice lactation support skills during their clinical rotations, and their primary resource on breastfeeding is often the course textbook. For an undergraduate nursing course, an innovative educational strategy was developed using a series of breastfeeding scenarios with the incorporation of animated avatars. Each scenario connected to a larger case study similar to a day in the life of a postpartum nurse dealing with breastfeeding situations on the hospital unit. Students were given a list of links and breastfeeding resources beyond the course textbook they could use to address the scenarios.

Nurse educators are constantly challenged to cover vast amounts of content in a limited time frame. This must be balanced with providing clinical experiences that give students an opportunity to apply knowledge learned in didactic courses. Maternal–child health courses must cover the full gamut of the perinatal period from preconception to postpartum. Students must learn skills for labor support, as well as postpartum care, including the support and promotion of breastfeeding. Despite the fact that breastfeeding is an important component of maternal–child nursing curriculum, breastfeeding support skills and knowledge of students has been found to be lacking (Freed, Clark, Harris, & Lowdermilk, 1996; Spear, 2006). Compounding this problem is the primary source of breastfeeding information a student might access is the required course textbook. Many of the maternal–child nursing textbooks have been found to be lacking in consistent and accurate information about breastfeeding (Phillipp, McMahon, Davies, Santos, & Jean-Marie, 2007).

In addition, the only opportunity students have to practice lactation support skills is during their clinical rotations. These rotations are often limited, and in rural settings, role modeling or access to a practicing lactation specialist are limited. The focus for this project was to provide students with an opportunity to practice application of breastfeeding support skills and use other breastfeeding resources to guide clinical lactation problem–solving situations.

Background

Computer technology has been integrated into many forms of education. The current generation of students has grown up in the digital environment and learns in different ways than prior generations (Brown, 2006). Today's generation of "digital natives" demand education via digital means (Milne, 2007; Skiba, 2007).

This paradigm shift has required teachers to enhance their educational strategies. However, integrating technology into teaching and learning in conjunction with traditional classroom lectures has been challenging (Lapadat, 2011). It not only requires the technological equipment but also involves the training of those that do not have experience in this new form of instruction. Today's nursing students are increasingly comfortable with the use of technology as part of their coursework. Many courses are delivered online, and the bulk of testing is given online to emulate the nursing licensure exam.

The Use of Avatars

A simplified model of an avatar is a three-dimensional (3-D) digital representation of a talking head that animates a human figure (Blake & Moseley, 2010). The facial features, hairstyle, and speech can be customized. Some have referred to them as animated pedagogical agents (Johnson, Rickel, & Lester, 2000), social models (Baylor,2009), virtual humans (Baylor & Kim, 2009), or embodied interface agents or avatars (Ma, Le, & Deng, 2011).

Bill Sheridan—Using Avatars to Innovate Education

The use of avatar talking heads has offered educators new ways to present information. Most educators have concentrated on the use of 3-D virtual environments, such as Second Life. Instead of using the virtual environments, Commendador and Chi (2013) designed avatar talking heads to teach case studies in a pediatric nursing class. The students were engaged and felt positive about this form of educational modality. By using the modality, the instructor can simply create an avatar scenario based on a case study and then make it available for students to access it online in self-paced and virtual synchronous way.

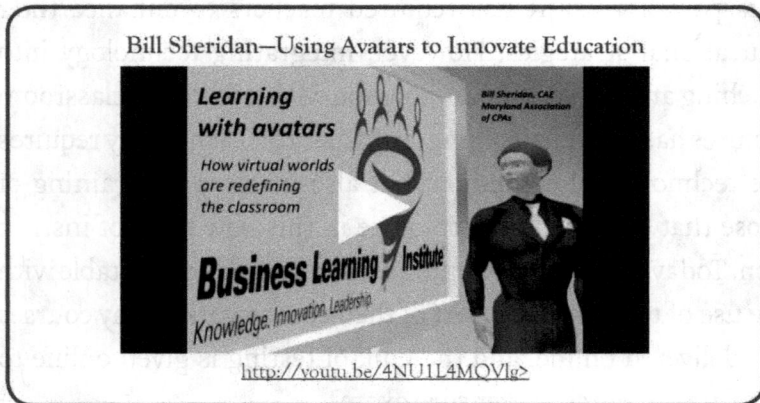

Bill Sheridan—Using Avatars to Innovate Education

Learning with avatars

How virtual worlds are redefining the classroom

Business Learning Institute
Knowledge. Innovation. Leadership.

Bill Sheridan, CAE
Maryland Association of CPAs

http://youtu.be/4NU1L4MQVlg>

Creating an Avatar

The creation of an avatar is simple with the use of a program such as SitePal (2003). The site allows users to create speaking avatars. One can either subscribe to a site for a monthly fee or pay an annual fee. The expense is based on the number of streams and features desired. Following the creation of the avatar, it can be published to web pages, email, PowerPoint, or Facebook.

The first step is to choose the type of avatar. One can choose either male or female from a variety of ethnicities. Generally, the upper body of the avatar is what the viewer sees. A background can also be selected, which will create the setting for the avatar. For example, if the avatar is designated to be a nurse, then the background could be a hospital unit. Or if the avatar is to be a patient in a hospital, a background resembling a hospital room can be chosen.

The second step is to create the text for the avatar to speak. This is typed into a dialogue box. One can preview and edit until the scenario is spoken as desired. The last step is the creation of the hyperlink or to publish the avatar to the desired site.

The Breastfeeding Avatar Assignment

The avatar assignment was created as a portion of a theory course for maternal–child nursing in a baccalaureate nursing program. Over a 2-year period, 60 students completed the assignment. The avatar assignment was posted on an online course delivery platform for the course. Each avatar was listed with a hyperlink on which students clicked and connected to http://www.sitepal .com/howitworks_B.

For this project, six avatars were created using SitePal. For each avatar, a breastfeeding case study scenario was developed based on the lactation consultant experiences of the faculty. Each scenario connects to a larger case study of a day in the life of a postpartum nurse dealing with breastfeeding situations on the unit. Three of the scenarios consisted of a nurse avatar giving report about breastfeeding patients. Three of the scenarios were situations involving a new mother or father on a postpartum unit of a hospital. Table 1 shows a list of the avatars and the focus of the scenario.

After viewing each avatar, the students were given one to three questions asking them to respond to the information they were given. The students were also given a list of links and breastfeeding resources beyond the course textbook they could use to address the scenarios. On a designated day, students brought their responses to the questions to class. During class, each avatar was replayed and the questions discussed and responded to by the students. Students were encouraged to share and add to the case study discussion with their clinical experiences. Students were given a pass/fail core based on completion of the questions, which were due prior to the class discussion. They were allowed to make corrections during the discussion.

Sample Scenarios

One of the nurse avatars was a postpartum nurse. Figure 1 shows the nurse avatar. For this scenario, the animated nurse avatar reports that an infant was taken to the nursery and given glucose water. Students were asked the following questions:

1. What are some possible rationales for taking the baby to the nursery for observation after the birth? Can you identify current evidence-based practice/policy for care of infants following delivery?

2. Why do you think the baby was given first sterile water and then glucose feedings in the nursery? Are there any contraindications to this practice?

3. What questions might you ask for more information from the reporting nurse?

Another scenario includes a young mother animated avatar who is complaining of sore nipples and an infant who wants to "nurse all the time." Figure 2 shows the avatar. Following the avatar, the students were asked:

1. What are some observations you would make in this situation?

2. How can you help the baby nurse on both sides?

Table 1. Summary of Breastfeeding Avatars	
Avatar	Breastfeeding Scenario
Postpartum nurse giving shift report	Overview of feeding issues on the unit including use of glucose water and nursery practices
Postpartum nurse responding to additional information requested by student and directed to father coming to nursing station	Address potential reasons for feeding difficulties and relationship to delivery
Father asking for help with infant and requesting bottle of formula	How to respond to a father's concerns including the use of formula
New mother discouraged and baby is sleepy	How to respond and encourage and assist a new mother
Postpartum nurse reporting on another mom	Causes and treatment for sore nipples
Postpartum mother with sore nipples	Important observations and how to assist

Project Efficacy

Breastfeeding is one of the most important preventative health practices a new mother can choose for herself and for her infant. For the novice nurse or nursing student, providing breastfeeding support is a major component of the job of the maternal–child nurse. Trying to incorporate all the aspects of the role of the maternal–child nurse is a challenge given the time constraints of a nursing course. There are many concepts that need to be taught that cannot be learned just by rote memorization. The challenge for educators is to prioritize and manage the important concepts. An even bigger challenge is engaging the student.

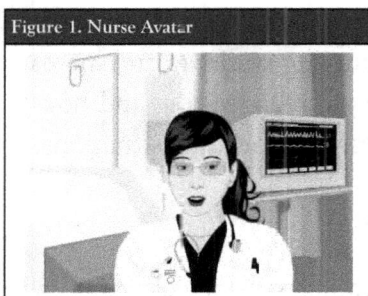
Figure 1. Nurse Avatar

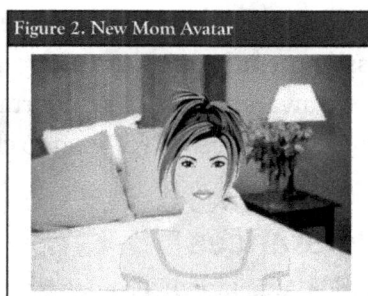
Figure 2. New Mom Avatar

The use of animated avatars proved to be successful using this online educational modality. Nurses have an influential role in supporting breastfeeding. In this educational project, the students were faced with multiple scenarios, which were similar as to what a nurse could expect on a busy obstetric unit. The students completed the online assignment, and in class, they were engaged and participated in the discussion of the possible responses.

The amount of effort the students put into answering their questions varied; however, many students researched the breastfeeding links for answers to the questions beyond what was expected. The case study scenarios allowed the students to practice critical thinking and apply it to the given scenarios. Learning is not just about acquiring knowledge and skills but applying it in practice. The students' education was augmented and supported with this educational modality. They gained new insights and new ways of doing things outside of the traditional textbook.

Implications for Practice

Using a virtual medium, such as avatars, allows educators to customize course assignments to specific curriculum. It is an effective way to link didactic course work to actual practice. Future breastfeeding scenarios could include mastitis, real or perceived milk supply, or other breastfeeding issues. This customizable assignment is one way to engage nursing students and increase their awareness of the importance of breastfeeding and how to access resources to respond to clinical breastfeeding situations.

References

Baylor, A. L. (2009). Promoting motivation with virtual agents and avatars: Role of visual presence and appearance. *Philosophical Transactions B, 364*, 3559–3565, http://dx.doi.org/10.1098/rstb.2009.0148

Baylor, A. L., & Kim, S. (2009). Designing nonverbal communication for pedagogical agents: When less is more. *Computers in Human Behavior, 25*, 450–457. http://dx.doi.org/101016/j.chb.2008.10.008

Blake, A. M., & Moseley, J. L. (2010). The emerging technology of avatars: Some educational considerations. *Educational Technology, 50*(2), 13–20.

Brown, J. (2006). *New learning environments in the 21st century: Exploring the edge.* Paper presented at the meeting of Forum for the Future of Higher Education, Cambridge, MA.

Commendador, K., & Chi, R. (2013). Comparative analysis of nursing students' perspectives toward avatar learning modality:

Gain pre-clinical experience via self-paced cognitive tool. *Journal of Interactive Learning Research, 24*(2), 151–166.

Freed, G. L., Clark, S. J., Harris, B. G., & Lowdermilk, D. L. (1996). Methods and outcomes of breastfeeding instruction for nursing students. *Journal of Human Lactation, 12*(2), 105–110. http://dx.doi.org/10.1177/089033449601200212

Johnson, W. L., Rickel, J. W., & Lester, J. C. (2000). Animated pedagogical agents: Face to face interaction in interactive learning environments. *International Journal of Artificial Intelligence in Education, 11*, 47–78.

Lapadat, J. (2011). Technologically mediated delivery in higher education: The margin as a site for change. In T. Bastiaens & M. Ebner (Eds.), *Proceedings of world conference on educational multimedia hypermedia and telecommunications 2011* (pp. 796–804). Chesapeake, VA: Association for the Advancement of Computing in Education. Retrieved from http://www.editlib.org/p/37958

Ma, X., Le, B. H., & Deng, Z. (2011, May). *Perceptual analysis of talking avatar head movements: A quantitative perspective.* Paper presented at the Proceedings of the SIGCHI Conference on Human Factors in Computing Systems, Vancouver, Canada. Retrieved from http://graphics.cs.uh.edu/publication /pub/2011_CHI_headMotionPerceptualAnalysis.pdf

Milne, A. J. (2007). *Entering the interaction age: Implementing a future vision for campus learning spaces.* Educause Review, 42(1), 12–31. Retrieved from http://connect.educause.edu/er

Philipp, B. L., McMahon, M. J., Davies, S., Santos, T., & Jean-Marie, S. (2007). *Breastfeeding information in nursing textbooks needs improvement.* Journal of Human Lactation, 23(4), 345–349. http://dx.doi.org/10.1177/0890334407307576

SitePal. (2003). *Oddcast.* Retrieved from http://www.sitepal.com/aboutus/

Skiba, D. (2007). Nursing education 2.0: Second life. *Nursing Education Perspectives, 29*(3), 156–157.

Spear, H. J. (2006). Baccalaureate nursing students' breastfeeding knowledge: A descriptive survey. *Nurse Education Today, 26*(4), 332–337. http://dx.doi.org/10.1016/j.nedt.2005.10.014

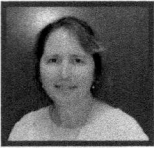

Jeanie Flood, PhD, RN, IBCLC, is an associate professor at University of Hawaii at Hilo School of Nursing. She has more than 20 years' experience caring for mothers and babies.

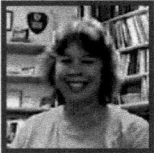

Kathleen Commendador, PhD, WHNP-BC, is a woman's health nurse practitioner with more than 20 years' experience caring for women. She is currently employed as an associate professor at University of Hawaii at Hilo School of Nursing.

USLCA

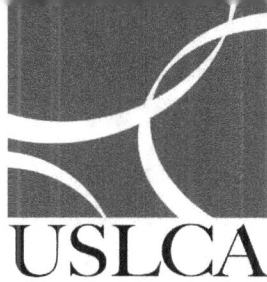

Standardizing Prenatal Breastfeeding Education in the Clinic Setting

Sherry L. Seibenhener, DNP, FNP-C, WHNP-BC

Leigh Minchew, DNP, RN, WHNP-BC

Keywords: breastfeeding, education, prenatal, provider, outcomes

The American Academy of Pediatrics recommends breastfeeding for the first 6 months of newborn life. Current research demonstrates women value the advice of obstetrical providers more so than that of family and friends. Unfortunately, there is often minimal to no breastfeeding education prenatally, and any education given may be fragmented, poorly timed, or influenced by provider experience. To improve consistency of breastfeeding education, a quality improvement project was developed and implemented in a local women's health clinic. This article discusses elements of the project to standardize prenatal breastfeeding education to support to the expecting mother and newborn.

Breastfeeding is a first step in health promotion for newborns. Healthy People 2020's goal of 81% of women initiating breastfeeding and 25% of those exclusively breastfeeding for up to 6 months reflects support for breastfeeding (Chung, Raman, Trikalinos, Lau, & Ip, 2008). The Joint Commission (TJC) demonstrated support of breastfeeding with Perinatal Core

Measure PC-05 Exclusive Breast Milk Feeding (United States Breastfeeding Committee, 2011) specifically focused on initiation and continuation of breastfeeding. Paralleling the American Academy of Pediatrics (AAP, 2012) recommendation, the Institute of Medicine (IOM, 2011b) released Recommendation 4-1 advising providers to encourage exclusive breastfeeding for at least the first 6 months of life. When TJC, AAP, and IOM recognize breast milk as the most beneficial food choice for newborns in the first 6 months, breastfeeding can be considered best practice for newborn nutrition.

The new practice standard for newborn nutrition presents providers the opportunity to promote breastfeeding in the clinic setting. A simple, strategic practice change is provider-based breastfeeding education during the prenatal period (Lin, Kuo, Lin, & Chang, 2008). Sadly, many providers lack depth in breastfeeding knowledge, leading to inconsistent or absent breastfeeding education (Chertok, Luo, Culp, & Mullett, 2011; Szucs, Miracle, & Rosenman, 2009).

Problem

Education is more effective when received in a timely manner and presented by someone knowledgeable on the topic (Watkins & Dodgson, 2010). When contemplating newborn feeding choices, women hold the opinions of their provider in higher regard than even family and friends (Vehid, Haciu, Vehid, Gokcay, & Bulut, 2009). However, if the provider does not educate and encourage breastfeeding, the mother has no other point of reference than family and friends. Vehid et al. (2009) illustrated women who receive prenatal breastfeeding education have improved attitudes, understanding, and skill with breastfeeding through the newborn's first 6 months of life and beyond. Unfortunately, providers caring for expecting women demonstrated a lack of interest, knowledge, or understanding of breastfeeding practices (Vehid et al., 2009). To that end, the Academy of Breastfeeding Medicine (ABM; ABM Protocol Committee, 2009) developed Clinical Protocol #19 to serve as a road map for practices to develop and enhance breastfeeding promotion in a clinic setting.

Literature Review

Searching CINAHL, the Cochrane Library, EBSCO, MEDLINE, and the National Guideline Clearinghouse for the time frame June 2008 through September 2013 collected evidence to identify breastfeeding practices, preferences, initiation and continuation, and barriers and facilitators encountered by expecting women and their providers. Inclusion criteria were full text articles, relevance to provider influence on breastfeeding initiation, interventions to optimize breastfeeding initiation and continuation, and breastfeeding education. Keywords included breastfeeding, breastfeeding, initiation, prenatal, education, preferences, and barriers. Articles included for final review consisted of two expert opinions, four qualitative surveys, three retrospective studies, three interventional studies, six systematic reviews, two case-control studies, and three randomized control trials.

Breastfeeding is a key in the growth and development of newborns, aiding mothers in development of parenting skills, enhancing maternal–newborn bonding, and facilitating maternal returns to healthy weights (Pate, 2009; Stuebe & Schwarz, 2010). Although evidence supports these benefits, barriers persist in initiation and continuation of breastfeeding (Ku & Chow, 2010; McKeever & Fleur, 2012; Silfverdal, 2011). A recurring theme in strategies to alleviate barriers and facilitate breastfeeding is provider-based education during the prenatal period (Lin et al., 2008).

Unfortunately, many women's health providers do not have strong breastfeeding knowledge and skill and compensate by using personal experience in place of current evidence, thereby repeatedly failing to provide consistent or accurate breastfeeding education (Chertok et al., 2011; O'Connor, Brown, & Lewin, 2011; Szucs et al., 2009). Reviewed literature supports the need for further research into breastfeeding practices, knowledge, skill, and attitudes of women's health providers and how these things influence breastfeeding initiation and continuation. Prenatal breastfeeding education was a noted strategy to maximize breastfeeding initiation and continuation (Kazemi & Ranjkesh, 2011).

The purpose of this article is to discuss the quality improvement project (QIP) for standardization of prenatal breastfeeding education to increase breastfeeding initiation, thereby improving quality outcomes for mothers and infants.

Intended Improvement

Quality should be evident in-patient care. Individuals committed to quality are in constant pursuit of excellence and continually look for ways to improve services. With Crossing the Quality Chasm (IOM, 2001a), an inherent need for quality in care has evolved. The QIP to standardize prenatal breastfeeding education incorporated IOM domains of timely, effective, and patient-centered care in pursuit of quality and excellence. Standardizing prenatal breastfeeding education encourages breastfeeding initiation and continuation. The overall project goal to standardize and initiate breastfeeding education during the prenatal period targeted the Healthy People 2020 benchmark for breastfeeding initiation (United States Breastfeeding Committee, 2013). As explained by Brenner and Buescher (2011), benefits achieved through breastfeeding are sufficient enough to mandate breastfeeding education so it becomes a quality clinical imperative.

Framework

Pender's (2011) health promotion model most closely aligned with elements of the QIP. Pender guides nursing practice to recognize patient-perceived influences on health promotion, provide counseling to patients, and promote healthy behaviors. Health promotion is imperative in optimizing outcomes and should be the heart of patient care. With promotion of healthy behaviors such as breastfeeding, nursing practice supports the patient in maximizing health and well-being.

The quality improvement model used to develop the QIP was the plan-do-study-act (Institute for Healthcare Improvement, 2013). Activities during the plan phase included a detailed literature review to identify evidence for best practice with prenatal breastfeeding education and strategies best suited to guide implementation of the QIP. Identified stakeholders in the QIP consisted of physicians, midlevel providers, nurses, expecting women, the significant other, and the newborn. In January 2014, 30 medical records were reviewed to determine the number of expecting patients that declared a feeding preference or had any propensity toward breastfeeding. Audits helped determine if, when, and how breastfeeding education was given during prenatal care.

The QIP lead developed 10 web-based training (WBT) modules for physician education, a classroom in-service for nurses, and a focus group for expecting women and their significant other. The do phase consisted of physician and nurse training, a focus group, and chart audits. The do phase will be discussed in further detail to follow. During the study phase, the QIP lead studied project results and disseminated findings to the identified stakeholders. The act phase came full circle, returning the QIP back to the planning phase to address identified shortcomings with the initial plan as well as looking toward sustaining quality improvement seen with successful changes.

Methods

Based on IOM (2011b), TJC (United States Breastfeeding Committee, 2011), ABM (ABM Protocol Committee, 2009), and Healthy People 2020 (Chung et al., 2008) recommendations, a QIP to standardize breastfeeding education in the clinic setting was developed and executed. The purpose was in accordance with IOM quality domains, serving to optimize health outcomes through breastfeeding initiation and continuation. Approval for the QIP was obtained from the institutional review board (IRB) and the clinic physician partnership.

Identified percentage change in breastfeeding initiation after prenatal education served to quantify project success, positively answering the QIP guiding question: "Will women who receive breastfeeding education during the prenatal period have higher rates of breastfeeding initiation and continuation through the infant's first 6 months of life as compared to women who do not receive prenatal education?"

Setting

The project was conducted in a women's health clinic that uses seven obstetricians, delivering approximately 1,400 babies annually (Lee Obstetrics & Gynecology, n.d.), and three gynecologists. Nonphysician medical staff includes 1 physician assistant, an ultrasound technician, 2 laboratory technicians, 12 nurses, a nurse manager, and 4 technicians.

Project Sample and Design

The QIP was a nonexperimental design with no control group used in implementation. Included in chart audits was a convenience sample of 30 females receiving care in the clinic, randomly selected from current and recently delivered obstetrical patients. Inclusion criteria were age (18–40 years), English-speaking, expecting, and literate. Exclusion criteria included preference for exclusive formula feeding after breastfeeding education was received, HIV or other medically contradictive barriers to breastfeeding, and surgically interrupted mammary functioning. Sample demographics can be seen in Table 1.

Table 1. Standardizing Prenatal Breastfeeding Education in the Clinic Setting Chart Audit 1 Data Comparison			
N = 30	January 2014	March 2014	May 2014
Age Range (years)	15–42	22–41	21–42
Ethnicity	White: 57%	White: 77%	White: 80%
	Black: 27%	Black: 17%	Black: 7%
	Asian: 13%	Asian: 3%	Asian: 10%
	Other: 3%	Other: 3%	Other: 3%
Feeding Type Initiated	Breast: 70%	Breast: 91%	Breast: 97%
	Formula: 27%	Formula: 9%	Formula 3%
	Both: 3%	Both: 0%	Both: 0%
Prenatal Documentation	Yes: 17%	Yes: 20%	Yes: 57%
	No: 83%	No: 80%	No: 43%

Project Implementation

Physician training commenced January 2014 with WBT modules focusing on strategies to increase breastfeeding rates, neonatal immunology and its association with breastfeeding, and management of breastfeeding dilemmas such as mastitis. Modules were administered and managed by the QIP lead. The clinic's practice manager was enlisted to maximize physician participation in the training.

A lunch and learn was used to deliver training to the clinic nursing staff at a date/time chosen to minimize conflict with clinic schedules. It was possible to capture staff during the workday, without detracting from work time, thereby optimizing staff participation in training.

A focus group was held to delve into the community mindset and awareness related to breastfeeding. Participants were volunteers from the clinic's obstetrical population and their preferred support person. The session was planned for February 2014, session held after clinic office hours, in the clinic practice site.

In March 2014, a chart audit was completed to evaluate postintervention breastfeeding initiation rates, providing information regarding breastfeeding education and initiation rates immediately after training was completed.

March audit data was then assessed against the preintervention January 2014 audit data.

Knowledge assessments were conducted at the completion of training in March 2014 for physician and nursing staff. The assessment consisted of 12 breastfeeding-related questions, presented in a 5-point Likert scale. The questions were structured to determine individual understanding and practice beliefs for both physician and nurse staff.

A final chart audit provided two data sets: The first determined if patients who initiated breastfeeding had continued breastfeeding at the time of their scheduled postpartum office visit, and the second revealed documented breastfeeding education, support, or interventional management provided by the physician or nurse staff.

Results

On January 14, 2014, seven obstetricians were assigned 10 WBT modules focused on breastfeeding. To track physician progress through the modules, the QIP ran weekly reports to determine percentage of module completion. Three physicians completed training by the second week of February. At the end of the project, one physician completed eight modules, one completed six modules, one completed a single module, and one physician never initiated module training.

In response to slow physician start, the QIP lead created and displayed a metric board showing physician completion rates for colleagues to see. Although the board fostered a healthy competition among providers, only a few stepped up their compliance. To solicit feedback regarding module content, applicability to practice, and method of training, an overview session was conducted for discussion and review.

On February 4, 2014, a lunch and learn was held for 12 registered and 1 practical nurse. The in-service provided basic breastfeeding knowledge and a script for use during patient interview, triage, and clinic childbirth education classes. An IBCLC provided clinical expertise and support for the in-service and ensuing questions. An additional incentive for nurses was the provision of continuing education credit.

On February 17, 2014, a focus group was conducted to identify layperson's knowledge and understanding of breastfeeding and why breastfeeding is important in maternal–infant health. Participants were members of childbirth education classes offered by the clinic.

Consent to participate was obtained from each group member. The session was completed in 45 minutes. Participants were shy to speak up; however, as the session progressed, expecting mothers became more outspoken and participation increased. Expectant mothers voiced desire for breastfeeding discussions in the office but felt that if they didn't initiate it, the discussion didn't happen. A small number of participants planned to attend breastfeeding classes at the local hospital to get more breastfeeding information.

An audit was completed on March 31, using the same process and data collection tool as the January audit. Thirty charts were randomly selected to determine the number of women who initiated breastfeeding, and any evidence of prenatal education as documented in the clinic record. Of the charts audited, 93% of women initiated breastfeeding, with 20% having breastfeeding preference and prenatal education documented. The data was then compared to initial findings from the January audit. Table 1 depicts data comparison among all audit findings.

Knowledge assessment surveys were hand distributed to seven obstetricians on March 25, 2014 with instruction to complete by March 28, 2014. A follow-up meeting was held April 28, 2014 to discuss findings from the March chart audits and physician surveys. During the discussion, five physicians stated they provide breastfeeding education to their patients but do not take the time to document the interaction. In addition, physicians reported making recommendations to attend breastfeeding classes yet again failed to capture this in documentation. Survey data was compiled and findings are shown in Table 2.

A final audit was conducted in two stages in May 2014. In one stage, charts of the delivered women used in the March 2014 audit were reviewed to determine breastfeeding continuation. The data point being if women who initiated breastfeeding after delivery were still breastfeeding at their postpartum evaluation.

Of the 27 women who initiated breastfeeding, 17 (63%) were still breastfeeding at that time.

Table 2. Posttraining Knowledge Assessment	% Strongly Disagree	% Agree	% Strongly Agree
1. Supplemental feeding is detrimental to the establishment of a good milk supply.	0%	67%	33%
2. A mother who believes her milk supply is not adequate should be encouraged to supplement with formula.	83%	0%	17%
3. Breastfeeding and formula feeding provide equal protection against illness in the newborn.	100%	0%	0%
4. The only way to truly breastfeed is for the newborn to nurse at the breast.	100%	0%	0%
5. Pacifiers do not influence breastfeeding patterns or success.	67%	33%	0%
6. If a woman develops mastitis, she should stop breastfeeding until the infection is cleared.	100%	0%	0%
7. The most common cause of painful breastfeeding is a poor latch.	16.5%	67%	16.5%
8. Breastfeeding exclusively for the first 6 months of life has been linked to improved health outcomes in the newborn.	0%	17%	83%
9. Breastfeeding is a skill that comes naturally to all women who have babies.	100%	0%	0%
10. As a healthcare provider, I have a responsibility to maintain knowledge and skills that support breastfeeding dyads.	0%	67%	33%
11. It is the recommendation of the American Academy of Pediatrics to initiate and maintain breastfeeding for at least the first 6 months of life.	0%	17%	83%
12. If a mother doesn't breastfeed for at least 12 weeks, there is no benefit to her or the newborn.	100%	0%	0%

The second stage of the audit identified practice change for breastfeeding education and documentation. As with the March 2014 audit, 30 patient charts were randomly selected for a review. In the May audit, there was a 43% increase in the documentation of feeding preference and a 36% increase in the documentation of breastfeeding education. Attendance rates to childbirth or lactation class increased by 23% and 27%, respectively (Figure 1). Data obtained post–project intervention was then prepared for dissemination to stakeholders in July 2014.

Discussion

In effort to follow ABM (ABM Protocol Committee, 2009), AAP (2012), IOM (2011b), TJC (United States Breastfeeding Committee, 2011), and Healthy People 2020 (Chung et al., 2008) recommendations, a QIP to standardize prenatal breastfeeding education was implemented in a local women's health clinic. Project planning and result dissemination was framed using Standards for Quality Improvement Reporting Excellence (SQUIRE) guidelines (Ogrinc et al., 2015).

Pre- and postintervention chart audits were performed to determine the influence provider education and support had on an expectant mother's newborn feeding preference. The March 2014 audit demonstrated poor increase in breastfeeding education and documentation of any education given. Physicians voiced recognition of the importance of education, yet actions did not follow suit. In response, the QIP lead met with the physician group to review Clinical Protocol #19 (ABM Protocol Committee, 2009) and strategize methods to aid in capturing education given with documentation. The second audit positively reflected the additional preparation and planning, as evidenced by an increase in documentation metrics and breastfeeding rates.

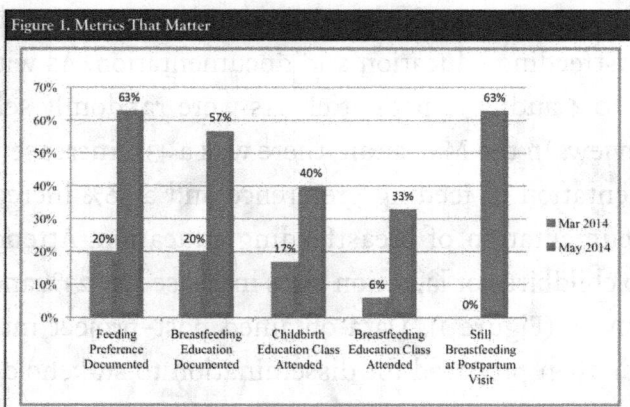

Figure 1. Metrics That Matter

An essential factor in project success is physician buy-in, recognizing the need to evaluate and change current practice because it relates to the delivery and documentation of prenatal breastfeeding education (O'Connor et al., 2011). The QIP lead's decision to use WBT modules for physician education was based on the idea that self-guided learning would encourage physicians to complete training in a timely manner. Unfortunately, forgoing a classroom setting prevented opportunity for social interaction, question and answer time, and positive peer pressure that promotes learner satisfaction (Jensen, Mondrup, Lippert, & Ringsted, 2009). Of interest was the fact that during face-to-face discussion, physicians voiced support and recognition of the need for breastfeeding training. However, only three of seven physicians completed all 10 WBT modules, with one not completing any. In consideration of the study by Olivieri, Knoll, and Arn (2009), the provision of continuing medical education credits may have promoted WBT compliance and completion.

When performing chart audits, the QIP lead identified an interesting data relevant to the patient's postpartum breastfeeding course. The delivering facility staffed a lactation department with two IBCLCs and four certified breastfeeding educators. Lactation staff was available to mothers 24/7 during hospitalization and by phone and support group after discharge. Mothers who breastfed in the hospital and maintained a relationship with lactation consultants and support group were more likely to continue breastfeeding, as evidenced by the 6-week postpartum continuation rates.

Limitations

The QIP was conducted in a private clinic providing obstetrical care in a moderate-sized community, resulting in a small sample that limited generalization of findings. In the same community, there are two other practices to which project findings may be of interest and applicable. To that end, additional breastfeeding projects should be devised, implemented, and evaluated. The project time frame was short, thereby limiting the depth in which each phase could be implemented and studied.

Excluding non-English-speaking patients also limits generalizability to the expecting population as a whole. According to the United States Census Bureau (2014), the population in 2012 was approximately 313,873,685 of which 16.9% were represented by Hispanic or Latino ethnicities. By 2050, it is estimated Hispanic or Latino cultures will represent 24% of the total population (Peterson-Iyer, 2008). In light of such statistics, inclusion of non-English-speaking patients is warranted. Another limitation involved physician training and the use of WBT modules as a sole training method. Physicians may have had too much autonomy to complete training in a timely manner. It is worth consideration to offer physicians education credits to incentivize completion. Also, face-to-face cumulative training to all providers at once with the opportunity for peer discussion of questions and concerns may facilitate physician training success.

Conclusion

Regardless of a woman's breastfeeding history, education is critical to breastfeeding initiation and continuation (ABM Protocol Committee, 2009). In addition, timing of education has been shown to play a key role in breastfeeding success. Introducing breastfeeding education during the prenatal period significantly improves breastfeeding initiation and continuation (Beake, Pellowe, Dykes, Schmied, & Bick, 2012).

Factors influencing feeding preference and intent include cultural practices, individual beliefs, and family recommendations (Vehid et al., 2009). Additional influencers are education, guidance, and support given to women by their providers. As providers, nurses are essential in identifying obstacles to breastfeeding success. Patient value placed on education creates an ideal opportunity for health promotion focusing on the maternal–infant pair. The QIP to standardize prenatal breastfeeding education establishes a foundation for all providers to cultivate practices promoting breastfeeding success, applicable across the pregnancy continuum.

References

Academy of Breastfeeding Medicine Protocol Committee. (2009). Clinical protocol number #19: Breastfeeding promotion in the prenatal setting. *Breastfeeding Medicine, 4*(1), 43–45. http://dx.doi.org/10.1089/bfm.2008.9982

American Academy of Pediatrics. (2012). Breastfeeding and the use of human milk. *Pediatrics, 129,* 600–603. Retrieved from https://www2.aap.org/breastfeeding/files/pdf/Breastfeeding2012ExecSum.pdf

Beake, S., Pellowe, C., Dykes, F., Schmied, V., & Bick, D. (2012). A systematic review of structured compared with nonstructured breastfeeding programmes to support the initiation and duration of exclusive and any breastfeeding in acute and primary health care settings. *Maternal & Child Nutrition, 8*(2), 141–161. http://dx.doi.org/10.1111/j.1740-8709.2011.00381.x

Brenner, M. G., & Buescher, E. S. (2011). Breastfeeding: A clinical imperative. *Journal of Women's Health, 20,* 1767–1773. http://dx.doi.org/10.1089/jwh.2010.2616

Chertok, I. R., Luo, J., Culp, S., & Mullett, M. (2011). Intent to breastfeed: A population-based perspective. *Breastfeeding Medicine, 6*(3), 125–129. Retrieved from http://online.liebertpub.com/doi/abs/10.1089/bfm.2010.0013

Chung, M., Raman, G., Trikalinos, T., Lau, J., & Ip, S. (2008). Interventions in primary care to promote breastfeeding: An evidence review for the U.S. preventative services task force. *Annals of Internal Medicine, 149*, 565–582.

Institute for Healthcare Improvement. (2013). *How to improve.* Retrieved from http://www.ihi.org/knowledge/Pages/ HowtoImprove/default.aspx

Institute of Medicine. (2001a). *Crossing the quality chasm: A new health system for the 21st century.* Retrieved from http://www. nationalacademies.org/hmd/~/media/Files/Report%20Files/2001/ Crossing-the-Quality-Chasm/Quality%20 Chasm%202001%20 %20report%20brief.pdf

Institute of Medicine. (2011b). *Recommendations: Healthy eating.* Retrieved from http://www.nationalacademies.org/hmd/ Reports/2011/Early-Childhood-Obesity-Prevention-Policies/ Recommendations.aspx

Jensen, M. L., Mondrup, F., Lippert, F., & Ringsted, C. (2009). Using e-learning for maintenance of ALS competence. *Resuscitation, 80,* 903–908. http://dx.doi.org/10.1016/j.resuscitation.2009.06.005. Epub 2009 Jul 1

Kazemi, H., & Ranjkesh, F. (2011). Evaluating the problems of mothers in exclusive and educational intervention for improving nutrition status in Iran. *HealthMED, 5*(6), 1517–1521. Retrieved from http://www.academia.edu/1324939/HealthMED_Journal_-_ Volume_5_No._6

Ku, C. M., & Chow, S. K. (2010). Factors influencing the practice of exclusive breastfeeding among Hong Kong Chinese women: A questionnaire survey. *Journal of Clinical Nursing, 19,* 2434–2445. http://dx.doi.org/10.1111/j.1365-2702.2010.03302.x

Lee Obstetrics & Gynecology. (n.d.). *Our mission.* Retrieved from http://www.leeobgyn.com

Lin, C.-H., Kuo, S.-C., Lin, K.-C., & Chang, T.-Y. (2008). Evaluating effects of a prenatal breastfeeding education programme on women with caesarean delivery in Taiwan. *Journal of Clinical Nursing, 17,* 2838–2845. http://dx.doi.org/10.1111/ j.13652702.2008.02289.x

McKeever, J., & Fleur, R. S. (2012). Overcoming barriers to babyfriendly status: One hospital's experience. *Journal of Human Lactation, 28,* 312–314. http://jhl.sagepub.com/content/early/2012/05/16/0890334412440627.abstract

O'Connor, M. E., Brown, E. W., & Lewin, L. O. (2011). An Internet-based education program improves breastfeeding knowledge of maternal-child healthcare providers. *Breastfeeding Medicine, 6,* 421–427. http://online.liebertpub.com/doi/ abs/10.1089/ bfm.2010.0061

Ogrinc, G., Davies, L., Goodman, D., Batalden, P., Davidoff, F., & Stevens, D. (2015). *SQUIRE 2.0 (Standards for Quality Improvement Reporting Excellence): Revised publication guidelines from a detailed consensus process.* Retrieved from http://qualitysafety.bmj.com/content/early/2015/09/10/bmjqs-2015-004411.full

Olivieri, J. J., Knoll, M. B., & Arn, P. H. (2009). Education format and resource preferences among registrants of a pediatricfocused CME website. *Medical Teacher, 31*(8), e333–e337. http://dx.doi.org/10.1080/01421590802650126

Pate, B. (2009). A systematic review of the effectiveness of breastfeeding intervention delivery methods. *Journal of Obstetric, Gynecologic, and Neonatal Nursing, 38,* 642–653. http://www.jognn.org/article/S0884-2175(15)30241-0/abstract

Pender, N. J. (2011). *The health promotion model manual.* Retrieved from https://deepblue.lib.umich.edu/bitstream/ handle/2027.42/85350/HEALTH_PROMOTION_MANUAL_Rev_5-2011.pdf

Peterson-Iyer, K. (2008). *Culturally competent care for Latino patients: An introduction.* Retrieved from https://www.scu.edu/ethics/ focus-areas/bioethics/resources/culturally-competent-care/ culturally-competent-care-for-latino-patients/

Silfverdal, S. A. (2011). Important to overcome barriers to translating evidence based breast-feeding information into practice. *Acta Paediatrica, 100,* 482–483. http://onlinelibrary.wiley.com/doi/10.1111/j.1651-2227.2011.02194.x/abstract

Stuebe, A. M., & Schwarz, E. B. (2010). The risks and benefits of infant feeding practices for women and their children. *Journal of Perinatology, 30*(3), 155–162. Retrieved from http://www.nature.com/jp/journal/v30/n3/full/jp2009107a.html

Szucs, K. A., Miracle, D., & Rosenman, M. B. (2009). Breastfeeding knowledge, attitudes, and practices among providers in a medical home. *Breastfeeding Medicine,* 4(1), 31–42. http://online.liebertpub. com/doi/abs/10.1089/ bfm.2008.0108?url_ver=Z39.88-2003&rfr_ id=ori%3Arid%3Acrossref.org&rfr_dat=cr_pub%3Dpubmed

United States Breastfeeding Committee. (2011). *Understanding The Joint Commission's perinatal care core measure set: A toolkit for hospitals in your state.* Retrieved from www.usbreastfeeding.org/d/do/150

United States Breastfeeding Committee. (2013). *Healthy people 2020: Breastfeeding objectives.* Retrieved from http://www. usbreastfeeding.org/LegislationPolicy/FederalPoliciesInitiatives/ HealthyPeople2020BreastfeedingObjectives/tabid/120/Default.aspx

United States Census Bureau. (2014). *State and county quick facts.* Retrieved from http://quickfacts.census.gov/qfd/states/00000.html

Vehid, H. E., Haciu, D., Vehid, S., Gokcay, G., & Bulut, A. (2009). A study of the factors affecting the duration of exclusive breastfeeding. *Nobel Medicus,* 5(3), 53–57. Retrieved from http://www.nobelmedicus.com/Content/1/15/53-57.pdf

Watkins, A. L., & Dodgson, J. E. (2010). Breastfeeding educational interventions for health professionals: A synthesis of intervention studies. *Journal for Specialists in Pediatric Nursing,* 15, 223–232. http://dx.doi.org/10.1111/j.1744-6155.2010.00240.x

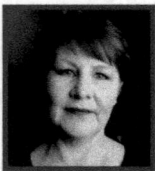

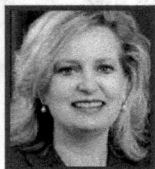

Sherry L. Seibenhener, DNP, FNP-C, WHNP-BC is an Assistant Professor in the Troy University College of Nursing in Montgomery, AL where she serves as coordinator of the ASN Program and Course Lead for Maternity Nursing theory and clinical courses. Dr. Seibenhener also serves as a committee member for DNP quality improvement projects. She has 26 years' nursing experience with over 16 years in OB/GYN nursing practice.

Leigh Minchew, DNP, RN, WHNP-BC is an Assistant Professor in the University of South Alabama's College of Nursing in Mobile, AL where she serves as coordinator of the Women's Health Nurse Practitioner Specialty Option. Dr. Minchew also serves as faculty advisor for DNP quality improvement projects. She has over 20 years' experience in OB/GYN nursing practice.

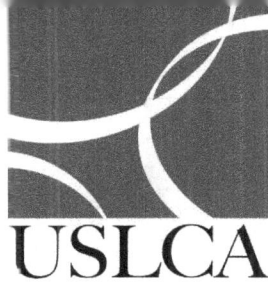

USLCA

Breastfeeding Knowledge and Intent to Breastfeed

An Integrative Review

Emily Lee, DNP, APRN, FNP-C, CLC

Joanie Jackson, DNP, APRN, FNP-BC

Keywords: breastfeeding, breastfeeding education, prenatal education, breastfeeding barriers, knowledge, healthcare provider

Objectives: *Identify, synthesize, and critically review research on common barriers to successful breastfeeding and ways healthcare providers can assist patients in overcoming the barriers.*

Methods: *A search of databases and citations for evidence-based research published from 2001 to 2015 was conducted. Forty-nine articles were reviewed with 22 articles being discussed.*

Results: *Three major themes were identified: (a) characteristics of breastfeeding education in the prenatal setting, (b) primary care interventions to promote breastfeeding, and (c) healthcare provider education on breastfeeding.*

Conclusions: *Findings of this review collectively suggest the need to increase breastfeeding rates among women in the United States. To achieve this, there is great significance*

placed on healthcare providers implementing interventions to promote breastfeeding, which subsequently requires improving healthcare provider knowledge and self-confidence on breastfeeding.

Breastfeeding is currently recognized as the ideal source of nutrition for most infants (American Academy of Pediatrics [AAP], 2012). The benefits of breastfeeding and the risks associated with formula feeding and early weaning from breastfeeding are well documented. Infants who are not breastfed are more likely to experience ear infections, incidents of diarrhea, and lower respiratory tract infections, and are at a greater risk of sudden infant death syndrome, diabetes, and obesity (AAP, 2012). Breastfeeding not only has numerous benefits to the infant but to the mother as well. Maternal benefits include a decreased incidence of developing breast and ovarian cancers, earlier return to pre-pregnancy weight, lessened postpartum bleeding, and quicker uterine involution (AAP, 2012).

In addition to the benefits to the mother and infant, breastfeeding has also been recognized as advantageous to society and the environment. Mothers who breastfeed their infants are sick less often, resulting in fewer work days missed because of illness. Breastfeeding does not need to be manufactured, and therefore, does not generate waste or pollution of the air. When compared with breast milk substitute, there is not a risk of contamination with breast milk, and it is continually at the precise feeding temperature (AAP, 2012). From an economic standpoint, a detailed pediatric cost analysis based on an Agency for Healthcare Research and Quality report concluded that if 90% of U.S. mothers would comply with the recommendation to breastfeed exclusively for 6 months, there would be a healthcare cost savings of $13 billion per year (Bartick & Reinhold, 2010).

According to the *Healthy People 2010* Objectives outcomes, the United States fell below the target on the proportion of infants who were breastfed ever, at 6 months, and at 1 year. The target was 75% for ever breastfed, 50% for still breastfeeding at 6 months, and 25% for still breastfeeding at 12 months. The United States also fell below the target for infants exclusively breastfed at both 3 and 6 months (Centers for Disease Control and Prevention [CDC], 2010). The *Healthy People 2020* Objectives, which focuses on increasing the proportion of infants who are breastfed, breastfed at 6 months, and breastfed at 12 months, have even higher targets. The target for ever breastfed has increased to 81.9%, the target for breastfeeding at 6 months has increased to 60.6%, and target for breastfeeding at 12 months has increased to 34.1%. Thus, it is critical for healthcare providers to consider why these goals have not been met in the past, how they can be met by the year 2020, and what the providers' role should be in assisting patients to successfully breastfeed (U.S. Department of Health and Human Services, 2010).

More women in the United States are becoming aware that breastfeeding is the ideal source of nutrition for their infants, but there continues to be a lack of knowledge about specific benefits of breastfeeding and the numerous risks associated with formula-feeding. Some mothers also lack the family and social support to breastfeed which many identify as a barrier to breastfeeding. The U.S. Department of Health and Human Services (USDHHS) has identified multiple barriers to breastfeeding, including social norms of bottle feeding, belief that larger babies are healthier, and embarrassment to breastfeed in public (USDHHS, 2011). Numerous lactation problems have also been identified as barriers: sore nipples, mastitis, engorged breasts, low milk supply, pain, difficulty with latch, and leaking milk. Navigating the difficulties of breastfeeding after returning to work is another common barrier. Possibly one of the most significant barriers is the lack of healthcare provider–related support and promotion of breastfeeding for the breastfeeding client (USDHHS, 2011). The purpose of this integrative review is to identify, synthesize, and critically review published research on the most common barriers to successful breastfeeding and the various ways healthcare providers can assist patients in overcoming the identified barriers during the prenatal period (USDHHS, 2011).

Method

The review of the literature began by searching the following online databases: the Cumulative Index to Nursing and Allied Health Literature (CINAHL), the Cochrane Library, Google Scholar, and PubMed/ MEDLINE. The terms, used alone and in combination, were breastfeeding, breastfeeding education, prenatal education, breastfeeding barriers, knowledge, and healthcare provider. Of the relevant studies identified, the Medical Subject Headings attached to them were also explored. After reviewing 49 abstracts, 27 studies were excluded for failure to meet inclusion criteria. The inclusion criteria consisted of only English language research studies conducted on adults in a developed country and those published between 2001 and 2015 in one of the previously mentioned databases. Exclusion criteria consisted of evaluation of the quality of the data, with lower quality evidence being excluded. The articles included in the review were further divided and categorized by common themes that emerged during the literature search.

Results

The three major themes developed during the literature search include (a) characteristics of breastfeeding education in the prenatal setting, (b) primary care interventions to promote breastfeeding, and (c) healthcare provider education on breast-feeding. Three articles discussed characteristics of breastfeeding education in the prenatal setting, 10 articles discussed primary care interventions to promote breastfeeding, and the remaining 10 articles discussed healthcare provider education on breast-feeding. Twenty-three articles that met selection criteria were retrieved and included in the review.

Theme 1: Characteristics of Breastfeeding Education in the Prenatal Setting

Information from three of the studies included in the review confirmed that healthcare provider support and encouragement had a positive effect on breastfeeding initiation and duration (Demirci et al., 2013; Holmes, 2013; Lu, Lange, Slusser, Hamilton, & Halfon, 2001). However, Demirci et al. (2013) reported that education on breastfeeding at the first prenatal visit was subpar, which contributed to a lack of breastfeeding education to patients by healthcare providers. The authors observed characteristics of first prenatal breastfeeding discussions between the patient and the healthcare provider which involved 69 healthcare providers and 377 patients (Demirci et al., 2013). Descriptive statistics were used to characterize the sample and frequency of breastfeeding discussions. The findings of this study revealed that discussions on breastfeeding were infrequent (29% of visits), brief (mean 39 seconds), and most often initiated by the healthcare providers in an ambivalent manner (Demirci et al., 2013).

In an article by Holmes (2013), the author indicated for successful breastfeeding, both patient education and preparation should begin before conception and occur during pregnancy. In the article, the author focused on reviewing the literature and summarizing the best available evidence surrounding the establishment of successful breastfeeding in the neonatal period.

The author began by summarizing interventions from the prenatal period that positively affect immediate breastfeeding outcomes in the postnatal period. In the article, the author indicated that many mothers make the decision to breastfeed their baby before even becoming pregnant, or early on in the first trimester of pregnancy, oftentimes before the initial prenatal visit (Holmes, 2013). Therefore, the author concluded that the influence of the primary healthcare provider early in the prenatal period on the decision to breastfeed is strong. The author also found that prenatal education was one of the most important interventions for increasing both breastfeeding initiation and duration (Holmes, 2013).

Lu et al. (2001) examined the influence of healthcare provider encouragement on breastfeeding among women of various social and ethnic backgrounds in the United States by evaluating the responses of 1,229 women with children younger than 3 years of age. Respondents were asked to recall whether their physicians or nurses had encouraged or discouraged them from breastfeeding, then the effects of healthcare provider encouragement was evaluated by multivariate logistic regression. More than 73% of the women reported having been encouraged by their healthcare providers to breastfeed; 74.6% of women who were encouraged initiated breastfeeding, compared with only 43.2% of those who were not encouraged (p , .001). Therefore, Lu et al. concluded that "provider encouragement significantly increases breastfeeding initiation" (p. 290), which in turn, increases the importance of the healthcare provider's time spent educating patients in the prenatal setting.

Theme 2: Primary Care Interventions to Promote Breastfeeding

Ten of the studies included in the review discussed effectiveness of interventions to promote breastfeeding in the primary care setting. There was a consensus in all 10 of the studies confirming that breastfeeding education and promotion had a positive effect on both initiation and duration of breastfeeding (Academy of Breastfeeding Medicine Protocol Committee, 2009; AAP, 2014; Betzold, Laughlin, & Shi, 2007; Chung, Raman, Trikalinos, Lau, & Ip, 2008; Dyson, McCormick, & Renfrew, 2005; Labarere et al., 2005; Lumbiganon et al., 2012; McLeod, Pullon, & Cookson, 2002; Nelson, 2012; Rempel & Moore, 2010). Dyson et al. (2005) completed a systematic review of the literature to evaluate the effectiveness of interventions that aim to encourage women to breastfeed and reported that "health education and peer support interventions can result in some improvements in the number of women beginning to breastfeed" (p. 2). Also, the authors discussed that greater increases are likely to result from needs-based, more informal repeat breastfeeding education sessions than common, formal antenatal sessions (Dyson et al., 2005).

In a similar article, a systematic review of the literature was conducted for the U.S. Preventive Services Task Force. Chung et al. (2008) suggested breastfeeding education and interventions are much more effective than typical prenatal care in increasing short- and long-term breastfeeding goals. Also, the authors discussed that a combination of both pre- and postnatal breastfeeding interventions, plus inclusion of nonprofessional support from the community, may be beneficial (Chung et al., 2008). A study by Rempel and Moore (2010) evaluated the effectiveness of a prenatal breastfeeding class developed and facilitated by peer "breastfeeding buddies," which included 54 expectant mothers who registered for the peer-led class, and 55 expectant mothers who registered for the nurse-led class. Authors' conclusions suggested that a prenatal class on breastfeeding led by peers was as effective as a traditional model of breastfeeding education and was a valued tool to promote and support successful breastfeeding.

Five of the articles related to this theme suggested that prenatal breastfeeding education along with management of breastfeeding situations were likely to increase the rates of initiation of breastfeeding and increase the duration of breastfeeding. McLeod et al. (2002) surveyed 490 women at different intervals during pregnancy and after giving birth. Data was collected on breastfeeding outcomes and experiences and was then analyzed using multiple logistic regressions. The authors determined that women were less likely to be exclusively breastfeeding at 6–10 weeks postpartum if they thought they required more breastfeeding information prior to delivery or had experienced problems while breastfeeding. This study represented the necessity for improvements in prenatal breastfeeding education (McLeod et al., 2002).

Three of the articles in this theme evaluated the effectiveness of breastfeeding interventions in the prenatal setting (Betzold et al., 2007; Labarere et al., 2005; Nelson, 2012) and were in agreement with previously stated findings from other studies that breastfeeding education in this critical prenatal setting has positive and significant impacts on breastfeeding. Two articles included in this theme were considered Level VII evidence because information was included from expert committees on the interventions to promote breastfeeding. One article was from the Academy of Breastfeeding Medicine Protocol Committee (2009) and included "Clinical Protocol Number 19." This protocol aimed to promote breastfeeding in the prenatal setting to impact breastfeeding success. Another article, from the AAP (2014) included Ten Steps to Support Parents' Choice to Breastfeed Their Baby. The steps included in this article was intended to aid healthcare providers in the education and support of parents in breastfeeding goals and decisions.

The final article included in this theme was a systematic review by Lumbiganon et al. (2012) which evaluated the effectiveness of antenatal breastfeeding education. Lumbiganon et al. concluded that it is not appropriate to recommend any specific antenatal breastfeeding education because of substantial methodological limitations and the observed effect sizes of the included studies were relatively small. The authors were aware of the importance of breastfeeding education but could not recommend a specific education tool and concluded the need for further randomized controlled trials with adequate power.

Theme 3: Healthcare Provider Education on Breastfeeding

The remaining 10 articles included in this review analyzed various forms of healthcare provider breastfeeding education in relation to breastfeeding promotion with patients. As previously indicated, a barrier is insufficient patient support of breastfeeding related to the lack of breastfeeding knowledge of healthcare providers. Increasing healthcare provider knowledge and self-efficacy has been shown to have a positive and substantial impact on breastfeeding rates and promotion (USDHHS, 2011).

Taveras et al. (2004) recognized clinicians' opinions and practices associated with continuation of exclusive breastfeeding using a prospective cohort study of lowrisk mother–newborn pairs. Of the 288 mothers who were breastfeeding at 4 weeks, 53% were exclusively breastfeeding at 12 weeks, even though clinicians reported limited time during postnatal visits to address breastfeeding problems. The authors concluded that clinicians' practices regarding supplementation of formula with healthy newborns, and opinions concerning the significance of breastfeeding guidance, are associated with the probability that mothers will continue exclusive breastfeeding. The authors went on to conclude that guidelines to enrich the clinicians' ability to address breastfeeding difficulties within the limits of busy practices could improve the healthcare provider's ability to support exclusive breastfeeding (Taveras et al., 2004).

Mellin, Poplawski, Gole, and Mass (2011) revealed how a formalized educational program and adherence to breastfeeding protocols can increase exclusivity of breastfeeding while also improving healthcare provider knowledge, comfort level, and attitudes about breastfeeding. The formalized breastfeeding education program included a breastfeeding protocol, a resource guide for the healthcare providers, and educational presentation sessions. This was a quasiexperimental study that included a survey of pre- and postimplementation measurements. The study sample included obstetricians, pediatricians, and nurses who interacted with breastfeeding mothers at a Level III Regional Perinatal (subspecialty care) Center averaging 3,500 births per year. The authors reported that healthcare providers showed increased levels of both knowledge and comfort with breastfeeding practices after completion of the education program. However, there were no statistically significant changes in the attitudes about breastfeeding of the healthcare providers included in the sample. There was, however, an increase in the obstetrical nurse's observation of breastfeeding after the educational intervention (Mellin et al., 2011).

Another article included in this theme was a synthesis of the literature to review intervention studies with a focus on increasing the breastfeeding knowledge, self-confidence, and supportive behaviors of healthcare providers. Watkins and

Dodgson (2010) reviewed 14 articles and concluded that "the emphasis breastfeeding educators and advocates have placed on issues surrounding the immediate postpartum period was evident in the reviewed studies" (p. 226). This finding emphasized the need for a more extensive approach to facilitating effective breastfeeding across settings and throughout the first year of the infant's life. The authors further concluded that interventions through education may be successful in transforming healthcare providers' understanding and changing maternal behavior.

In an article by Bass (2015), the author suggested that pediatricians need to be both knowledgeable about breastfeeding and skilled in management of breastfeeding clients so that healthcare providers can advocate for breastfeeding in their practice. The author went on to state that with breastfeeding knowledge, healthcare providers can provide necessary anticipatory guidance and support to breastfeeding mothers and their infants. A 2012 statement by the AAP emphasized that healthcare providers should advocate for breastfeeding and be able to fully manage breastfeeding clients. Lack of healthcare provider knowledge, skills, and time during visits have all been cited as barriers to breastfeeding. The author also suggested that healthcare provider education programs could increase the exclusivity and duration of breastfeeding and decrease associated problems (Bass, 2015).

Five of the nine studies included in this theme examined the effects of an educational intervention on healthcare provider breastfeeding knowledge. Feldman-Winter et al. (2010) conducted a controlled trial of 417 residents using the "Residency Curriculum" developed by the AAP (AAP, 2010). The authors concluded that a breastfeeding course for residents in pediatrics, family medicine, and obstetrics and gynecology enhanced knowledge, practice patterns, and confidence in both breastfeeding management and exclusive breastfeeding. Hillenbrand and Larsen (2002) completed a similar study of 49 pediatric residents using an interactive multimedia curricular intervention to increase knowledge about common lactation issues and concluded that "not only breastfeeding knowledge and confidence, but most importantly clinical behaviors of pediatric residents can be enhanced through innovative educational opportunities" (p. 1). The authors suggested that proper guidance and management for breastfeeding mothers might contribute to an increase in the duration of breastfeeding. Two similar studies also looked at the effectiveness of interactive and web-based education programs for healthcare providers in efforts to increase breastfeeding knowledge (Kronborg, Vaeth, Olsen, & Harder, 2007; O'Connor, Brown, & Lewin, 2011). All authors concluded that the programs in the studies improved breastfeeding knowledge and had implications to improve breastfeeding rates and duration (Kronborg et al., 2007; O'Connor et al., 2011).

A study by Bonuck, Trombley, Freeman, and McKee (2005) was conducted to determine whether an individualized, prenatal and postnatal, lactation consultant intervention resulted in increased cumulative intensity of breastfeeding. This was a randomized, nonblinded, controlled trial that included 304 women. The authors concluded that the intervention was appropriate to increase breastfeeding duration and intensity. This study included lactation consultants, but similar interventions could be used with other healthcare providers (Bonuck et al., 2005).

Finally, a review by Chen, Johnson, and Rosenthal (2012) examined the association between breastfeeding duration and sources of education about breastfeeding and breast pumps. The authors analyzed data from the Infant Feeding Practices

Survey II (CDC, 2012) composed of 2,586 participants. This study was unusual because it resulted in a "negative association between longer breastfeeding duration and receiving breast pump education from a physician/physician assistant" and a "positive association between longer breastfeeding duration and receiving breastfeeding education from classes/ support group while receiving breast pump education from friends/relatives" (p. 1421). The authors went on to conclude that the negative association could likely have been because of the limited time and resources of clinical practice but could also have specified a need for more consistent preparation for healthcare providers who provided breastfeeding and/or breast pump education (Chen et al., 2012).

Discussion

Information from the literature review articles supported not only a need to increase breastfeeding rates but also a need for healthcare providers to implement interventions into practice in the prenatal period to promote breastfeeding. This, in turn, may help women overcome the aforementioned common barriers to breastfeeding. Although there is importance for healthcare providers to implement breastfeeding promotion, providers continue to lack the appropriate knowledge and skill set necessary to successfully promote breastfeeding through patient education and clinical practice.

The literature review articles were comparable in that breastfeeding promotion and support prenatally could significantly improve the number of women who initiate and then continue exclusive breastfeeding. Some authors in this review analyzed several educational tools, all of which were successful in increasing knowledge and self-confidence of healthcare providers. The educational tools were effective in overcoming the breastfeeding barrier which relates to a lack of healthcare provider knowledge in breastfeeding promotion and support. The articles included in this review emphasized the importance of educating healthcare providers regarding the significance of breastfeeding promotion and how to manage common breastfeeding problems. The commonalities of the articles were the skills, knowledge, and self-efficacy necessary for providers to adequately educate and support breastfeeding clients.

There are significant implications for practice and application of the educational tools discovered in this review, and as a result, healthcare providers can acquire skills and gain knowledge. It is proposed that once healthcare providers are more knowledgeable and confident in promoting breastfeeding, primary care interventions such as prenatal breastfeeding education and promotion can better facilitate mothers in achieving breastfeeding goals and overcoming common breastfeeding barriers. Therefore, breastfeeding rates could continue to increase once mothers are adequately educated and continually supported throughout their breastfeeding journey.

References

Academy of Breastfeeding Medicine Protocol Committee. (2009). Clinical protocol number #19 Breastfeeding promotion in the prenatal setting. *Breastfeeding Medicine*, 4, 43–45.

American Academy of Pediatrics. (2010). *Breastfeeding residency curriculum.* Retrieved from http://www2.aap.org/breastfeeding/curriculum/

American Academy of Pediatrics. (2012). *Breastfeeding and the use of human milk.* Retrieved from http://www2.aap.org/ breastfeeding/files/pdf/Breastfeeding2012ExecSum.pdf

American Academy of Pediatrics. (2014). *Ten steps to support parents' choice to breastfeed their baby.* Retrieved from https://www2.aap.org/breastfeeding/files/pdf/tenstepsposter.pdf

Bartick, M., & Reinhold, A. (2010). The burden of suboptimal breastfeeding in the United States: A pediatric cost analysis. *Pediatrics, 125*(5), e1048–e1056. Retrieved from http://pediatrics. aappublications.org/content/early/2010/04/05/ peds.2009-1616. short

Bass, P. (2015). *Evidence-based support for breastfeeding.* Retrieved from http://contemporarypediatrics.modernmedicine. com/contemporary-pediatrics/news/evidence-based-supportbreastfeeding?page=full

Betzold, C., Laughlin, K., & Shi, C. (2007). *A family practice breastfeeding education pilot program: An observational, descriptive study. International Breastfeeding Journal, 2,* 4.

Bonuck, K., Trombley, M., Freeman, K., & McKee, D. (2005). Randomized, controlled trial of a prenatal and postnatal lactation consultant intervention on duration and intensity of breastfeeding up to 12 months. *Pediatrics, 116,* 1413–1426. Retrieved from http://pediatrics.aappublications.org/content/116/6/1413.long

Centers for Disease Control and Prevention. (2010). *Healthy People 2010.* Retrieved from http://www.cdc.gov/nchs/healthy_people/ hp2010.htm

Centers for Disease Control and Prevention. (2012). *Infant Feeding Practices Study II and its year six follow-up.* Retrieved from http://www.cdc.gov/breastfeeding/data/ifps/index.htm

Chen, P., Johnson, L., & Rosenthal, M. (2012). Sources of education about breastfeeding and breast pump use: What effect do they have on breastfeeding duration? An analysis of the Infant Feeding Practices Survey II. *Maternal Child Health Journal, 16,* 1421–1430.

Chung, M., Raman, G., Trikalinos, T., Lau, J., & Ip, S. (2008). Interventions in primary care to promote breastfeeding: An evidence review for the U.S. Preventive Services Task Force. *Annals of Internal Medicine, 149,* 565–582. Retrieved from http://annals.org/article.aspx?articleid=743317

Demirci, J., Bogen, D., Holland, C., Tarr, J., Rubio, D., Li, J., . . . Chang, J. (2013). Characteristics of breastfeeding discussions at the initial prenatal visit. *Obstetrics and Gynecology, 122,* 1263–1270.

Dyson, L., McCormick, F. M., & Renfrew, M. J. (2005). *Interventions for promoting the initiation of breastfeeding.* Retrieved from http://onlinelibrary.wiley.com/doi/10.1002/14651858.CD001688.pub2/abstract;jsessionid=B0CA62E1E350F68AEF9D99628202AD16.f02t02

Feldman-Winter, L., Barone, L., Milcarek, B., Hunter, K., Meek, J., Morton, J., . . . Lawerence, R. (2010). Residency curriculum improves breastfeeding care. *Pediatrics, 126,* 289–297.

Hillenbrand, K., & Larsen, P. (2002). Effect of an educational intervention about breastfeeding on the knowledge, confidence, and behaviors of pediatric resident physicians. *Pediatrics, 110,* 1–7.

Holmes, A. (2013). Establishing successful breastfeeding in the newborn period. *Pediatric Clinics of North America, 60*(1), 147–168.

Kronborg, H., Vaeth, M., Olsen, J., & Harder, I. (2007). Health visitors and breastfeeding support: Influence of knowledge and self-efficacy. *European Journal of Public Health, 18,* 283–288.

Labarere, J., Gelbert-Baudino, N., Ayral, A., Duc, C., Berchotteau, M., Bouchon, N., . . . Pons, J. (2005). Efficacy of breastfeeding support provided by trained clinicians during an early, routine, preventive visit: A prospective, randomized, open trial of 226 mother-infant pairs. *Pediatrics, 115,* e139–e146. Retrieved from http://pediatrics.aappublications.org/ content/115/2/e139

Lu, M., Lange, L., Slusser, W., Hamilton, J., & Halfon, N. (2001). Provider encouragement of breast-feeding: Evidence from a national survey. *Obstetrics and Gynecology, 97*(2), 290–295.

Lumbiganon, P., Martis, R., Laopaiboon, M., Festin, M., Ho, J., & Hakimi, M. (2012). Antenatal breastfeeding education for increasing breastfeeding duration. *Cochrane Database of Systematic Reviews, 12,* CD006425.

McLeod, D., Pullon, S., & Cookson, T. (2002). Factors influencing continuation of breastfeeding in a cohort of women. *Journal of Human Lactation, 18,* 335–343.

Mellin, P., Poplawski, D., Gole, A., & Mass, S. (2011). Impact of a formal breastfeeding education program. *American Journal of Maternal Child Nursing, 36*(2), 82–88.

Nelson, A. (2012). A meta-synthesis related to infant feeding decision making. *American Journal of Maternal Child Nursing, 37*(4), 247–252.

O'Connor, M., Brown, E., & Lewin, L. O. (2011). An internetbased education program improves breastfeeding knowledge of maternal-child healthcare providers. *Breastfeeding Medicine, 6*, 421–427.

Rempel, L., & Moore, D. C. (2010). Peer-led prenatal breast-feeding education: A viable alternative to nurse-led education. *Midwifery, 28*, 73–79.

Taveras, E., Li, R., Grummer-Strawn, L., Richardson, M., Marshall, R., Rêgo, V., . . . Lieu, T. (2004). Opinions and practices of clinicians associated with continuation of exclusive breastfeeding. *Pediatrics, 113*, e283–e290.

U.S. Department of Health and Human Services. (2010). *Healthy People 2020*. Retrieved from http://www.healthypeople.gov/2020/default.aspx

U.S. Department of Health and Human Services. (2011). *The surgeon general's call to action to support breastfeeding. Washington, DC: U.S. Department of Health and Human Services*, 1–100. Retrieved from http://www.surgeongeneral.gov/library/calls/breastfeeding/calltoactiontosupportbreastfeeding.pdf

Watkins, A., & Dodgson, J. (2010). Breastfeeding educational interventions for health professionals: A synthesis of intervention studies. *Journal for Specialists in Pediatric Nursing, 15*(3), 223–232.

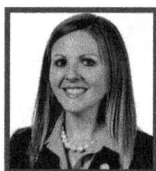

Emily Lee, DNP, APRN, FNP-C, CLC, is an instructor in nursing at the Whitson-Hester School of Nursing at Tennessee Technological University. Emily is passionate about breastfeeding and breastfeeding promotion. Sherecently completed her Doctor of Nursing Practice (DNP) degree in 2015 and her DNP project focused on increasing breastfeeding knowledge and confidence in healthcare providers. Emily became a certified lactation counselor during her doctoral studies as well.

Joanie Jackson, DNP, APRN, FNP-BC, is an assistant professor and DNP: Nursing Program Coordinator at The University of Tennessee at Chattanooga School of Nursing. Joanie began a career in academia in 2011 at UTC. Joanie graduated with a DNP (with a Forensic concentration) in 2008 and her practice experience, before coming to academia, has been in inpatient clinical patient safety and sexual assault.

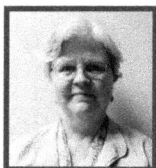

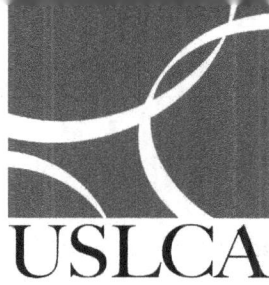

The Effect of an International Board Certified Lactation Consultant in the Pediatric Primary Care Setting on Breastfeeding Duration and Exclusivity During the First Year of Life

Cynthia A. Morris, DNP, RN, IBCLC, RLC

Judith L. Gutowski, BA, IBCLC, RLC

Keywords: breastfeeding support, pediatrician, infant, breastfeeding, outpatient setting, International Board Certified Lactation Consultant

Despite widely documented evidence that supports breastfeeding throughout the first year of life, many mothers quit breastfeeding earlier than intended. This retrospective review examined the effect of an International Board Certified Lactation Consultant (IBCLC) in the pediatric primary care setting on breastfeeding duration and exclusivity rates. In this study, access to an IBCLC in the pediatric primary care setting increased the odds of mothers breastfeeding longer than mothers who did not have such access. Neither term gestation nor previous history of childbirth affected the like-

lihood of mothers exclusively breastfeeding for 4–6 months or continuing breastfeeding for at least 1 year. Increasing maternal age did not increase the odds of exclusively breastfeeding until 4–6 months but did increase the odds of continuing to provide some breast milk for at least 1 year. The presence of an IBCLC in this setting was associated with increased breastfeeding duration, even among women who had no direct interaction with the consultant. Integrating an IBCLC into the pediatric primary care setting may be a viable option to increase breastfeeding duration and exclusivity rates.

The effort to increase breastfeeding initiation in the United States has been successful. This is evidenced by the fact that national breastfeeding initiation rates have risen steadily from 60% in 1995 to 76.9% in 2012 (Centers for Disease Control and Prevention [CDC], 2012; McDowell, Wang, & Kennedy-Stephenson, 2008). Unfortunately, efforts to enable women to follow through with infant feeding recommendations have fallen short. In that same time, breastfeeding until 6 months of age has only increased by 4.4% (CDC, 2012; Ryan, Wenjun, & Acosta, 2002).

The greatest decline in breastfeeding occurs among infants 2–6 weeks of age (Bonuck, Trombley, Freeman, & McKee, 2005). Hamlyn, Brooker, Oleinikova, and Wands (2002) reported that 87% of mothers who quit breastfeeding within 6 weeks of birth would have liked to continue breastfeeding longer. Odom, Li, Scanlon, Perrine, and Grummer-Strawn (2013) noted that 60% of mothers who quit breastfeeding before they desired did so because of concerns over breastfeeding difficulties, infant nutrition and weight, illness or need for medications, or the effort associated with pumping milk.

It has been well illustrated that continued outpatient support is necessary to improve breastfeeding duration and exclusivity rates (Castrucci, Hoover, Lim & Maus, 2007; Thurman & Allen, 2008; Wagner, Chantry, Dewey, & Nommsen-Rivers, 2013).

Unfortunately, many healthcare providers have not received adequate training to assess breastfeeding problems, provide support, and facilitate effective lactation management (Dodgson & Tarrant, 2007; Moore & Coty, 2006; Osband, Altman, Patrick, & Edwards, 2011). International Board Certified Lactation Consultants (IBCLCs) are healthcare professionals who have specialized in the clinical management of breastfeeding. They invest many hours in academic preparation and under direct clinical supervision to learn strategies to solve breastfeeding problems and to educate and support families and healthcare professionals (United States Department of Health and Human Services, 2011). IBCLCs are specifically trained to be an integral member of the healthcare team, providing a medically necessary service for breastfeeding women and their children (Gutoswki, Walker, & Chetwynd, 2012).

Many studies have examined and reported the positive effect of inpatient IBCLC services on breastfeeding initiation, duration, and exclusivity rates (Francis-Clegg & Francis, 2011; Lewallen et al., 2006; Mannel & Mannel, 2006). However, there is limited research which examines the effect of postpartum interactions with an IBCLC in the primary care setting on both breastfeeding duration and exclusivity. The purpose of this study is to address existing gaps in the literature as to the value of integrating IBCLCs into the primary care setting.

Method

This study was conducted as a retrospective chart review in a suburban southwestern Pennsylvania pediatric practice. The electronic medical record (EMR) of newborns admitted to the practice were reviewed for a 9-month period prior to hiring an IBCLC (pre-IBCLC group) and for a 9-month period after her integration into the office setting (IBCLC available group [IBCLC-A]). The IBCLC was available in the pediatric office 3 days each week. She offered face-to-face consultative services and support via telephone or email for all breastfeeding mothers who used this practice for medical care of their child.

The charts of 542 newborns admitted to the practice during the stated time were examined for feeding method at the initial well-child visit. Inclusion criteria for this study were infants who were breastfeeding or receiving breast milk at the initial visit to this pediatric practice. The initial visit must have occurred when the child was between 2 and 14 days of age. Excluded from this review were infants who were older than 2 weeks of age at first contact with this pediatric practice and infants in which the feeding method was not recorded in the progress notes at the initial visit. Initially, 332 infants (166 in each group) met inclusion criteria for this study.

Procedure

The physician progress notes of each breastfeeding infant included in the study were reviewed for recorded feeding methods at the well-child visits during the first year of life. These visits typically occurred at 1, 2, 4, 6, 9, and 12 months of age. Feeding methods at each defined interval were recorded as exclusively breast milk, breast and nonhuman milk, nonhuman milk, or breast milk plus foods. The World Health Organization defines exclusive breastfeeding as no food or drink other than breast milk. Predominate breastfeeding applies to infants who are receiving water, sugar water, and/or fruit juice in addition to breastfeeding. These infants are fed no other food-based fluid (Noel-Weiss, Boersma, & Kujawa-Myles, 2012).

For this review, exclusive breastfeeding and predominate breastfeeding were both coded as breastfeeding. Infants who are fed formula/nonhuman milk in addition to their consumption of breast milk were recorded as breast and nonhuman milk feeding. Children who were fed no breast milk but received formula or other nonhuman milk were classified as nonhuman milk feeding. Children who had started receiving solid/semi-solid foods but continued to drink only human milk were recorded as breastfed plus foods.

Information was also collected from each EMR regarding maternal age, previous history of childbirth, and the infant's gestational age at birth. Gestational age was recorded as either term status (38 weeks and older) or late preterm status (34–37 weeks). The effect of these variables on breastfeeding duration and exclusivity were examined in addition to the variable of access to an IBCLC.

The length of exclusive breastfeeding represents the latest period in which the mother reported having fed only human milk to her infant. Situations in which the mother fed her infant nonhuman milk but later returned to feeding only breast milk were recorded as to the latest date in which the mother reported that her infant had consumed nothing but human milk. Duration of any breastfeeding was based on the latest reported period during which the mother recounted providing any human milk, not preceded by any periods in which it was stated that no breast milk was provided.

Statistical Analysis

Of the 332 infant charts which met the inclusion criteria, 76 were missing variables which were of interest in this study. The variables were missing because of a wide range of circumstances such as physician not recording feeding method, child not attending a well-child visit, and birth hospital not recording maternal age or gestational age. Most missing values were either feeding status at one or more observation window (35 infant records) or maternal age (25 infant records).

To examine if there were differences between the groups in the proportion of missing feeding status windows, a chi-square analysis was performed. The pre-IBCLC group had 15 infant records with missing feeding status observations. The IBCLC-A group had 20. It was determined that there was no relationship between the two groups missing data ([N 5 332] 5 .511, p 5 .47).

Maternal age was not available for collection in 17 cases in the pre-IBCLC group and 8 cases in the IBCLC-A group. This variable was usually missing because of the birth hospital not including it on the newborn discharge summary. A chi-square analysis of the full data set indicated that there was no significant difference between the two groups missing variable of maternal age ([N 5 332] 5 2.77, p 5 .10).

Because of the complete randomness of the missing information, complete case analysis was implemented.

Table 1. Recoded Duration of Exclusive Breastfeeding				
Group	Infants Fed Breast Milk at Initial Well-Child Visit	Infants Supplemented Prior to the 1-Month Visit	Infants Exclusively Receiving Breast Milk at 1- to 2-Month Visit	Infants Exclusively Receiving Breast Milk at 4- to 6-Month Visit
Pre-IBCLC	120	47.5% (57)	52.5% (63)	21.7% (26)
IBCLC-A	136	41.2% (56)	58.9% (80)	33.1% (45)

Note. IBCLC = International Board Certified Lactation Consultant; IBCLC-A = International Board Certified Lactation Consultant available group.

The data sets' missing study variables were removed from further analysis. The final data set consisted of 256 patients, 120 in the pre-IBCLC group and 136 in the IBCLC-A group.

Various statistical analyses were performed on the remaining data sets. Initially, we used both student's t test and chi-square testing to ensure the independent variables of maternal age, gestational age, and previous history of childbirth did not differ based on the experimental group. We then compared the percentage rates of mothers in each group who reported exclusive breastfeeding of up to 6 months and continued provision of any breast milk up to 1 year.

Multinomial and binary logistic regressions were performed to determine which of the study variables had an effect on breastfeeding duration and exclusivity during the first year of life. Prior to conducting a multinomial logistic regression on variables which effect exclusive breastfeeding, the groups were recoded to provide a more readily interpretable and meaningful outcome variable. The data was recoded to reflect mothers who provided supplementation during the first month (o months of exclusive breast milk), 1–2 months of exclusive breast milk, or 41 months of exclusive breast milk (Table 1).

Because 12 months was the target date for duration of any breastfeeding, the data was recoded to reflect breastfeeding for 1 year versus less than 1 year prior to performing a binary logistic regression. Lastly, a binary logistic regression analysis was conducted predicting any breastfeeding at 12 months among women in the IBCLC-A group who did not interact with the lactation consultant. Any data set in which the mother had contact with the IBCLC via visits, emails, or phone calls was excluded from this analysis.

Results

Sample

The sample was significantly homogeneous (98.4% White). The average maternal age was 29.23 years (SD 5 5.12) and most had private health insurance (72.3%). The population was evenly split between first time mothers (49.6%) and mothers who had at least one previous delivery (50.4%). Most of the infants were of term status (85.5%) with only 14.5% delivered between 34 and 37 weeks gestation (late preterm).

The analyses revealed there were no significant differences in the independent variables between the experimental groups.

Maternal age was found to be normally distributed and to not significantly differ between the pre-IBCLC and IBCLC-A groups (p 5 .48). History of previous childbirth provided appropriate distribution for analysis and there was no observed differences between the two groups (p 5 .54). Term status also exhibited appropriate distribution for analysis and demonstrated no difference in proportions between experimental groups (p 5 .40).

Exclusive Breastfeeding Rates

It was evident that many mothers found the need to supplement with formula during the first month of life. Although 47.5% of mothers in the pre-IBCLC group supplemented with artificial baby milk during the first month of life, only 41.2% of the IBCLC-A group deemed it necessary. It was noted at each well-child visit observation window that women who had access to an IBCLC were more successful at the goal of exclusive breastfeeding than women in the pre-IBCLC group (Table 2).

Mothers who had access to an IBCLC had odds of 1.75 times greater than mothers in the pre-IBCLC group of exclusively breastfeeding until 4–6 months of age as compared to 0 month (p 5 .073). Similarly, mothers in the IBCLC-A group were 1.83 times more likely than mothers in the pre-IBCLC group to be exclusively breastfeeding to 4–6 months as compared to 1–2 months (p 5 .080). These differences were only marginally significant. Maternal age, previous history of child birth, and term status was not found to be statistically predictive of exclusive breastfeeding behavior (Table 3).

Table 2. Duration of Exclusive Breastfeeding Based on Well-Child Visits					
Group	Infants Fed Any Breast Milk at Initial Visit	Infant Reported to Be Exclusively Breastfed at Specified Well-Child Visit Interval			
		1-Month Visit	2-Month Visit	4-Month Visit	6-Month Visit
Pre-IBCLC	120	52.5% (63)	36.7% (44)	21.7% (26)	5.0% (6)
IBCLC-A	136	58.8% (80)	47.8% (65)	33.1% (45)	8.8% (12)

Note. IBCLC = International Board Certified Lactation Consultant; IBCLC-A = International Board Certified Lactation Consultant available group.

Duration of Any Breastfeeding

Access to an IBCLC was significantly predictive of continued breastfeeding for at least 1 year. Although the rates for providing any breast milk were only slightly higher for the IBCLC-A group during the first few months of breastfeeding, a much greater difference became apparent in the second half of the first year. Refer to Table 4.

In the IBCLC-A group, 26.5% (n 5 36) were still providing breast milk at the 12-month well-child visit. Only 14.2% (n 5 17) of mothers in the pre-IBCLC continued to provide breast milk until the same interval. Table 5 displays the results of a binary logistic regression performed to predict differences between the two groups. Mothers in the IBCLC-A group were 2.15 times more likely to be providing some breast milk for a year than were mothers in the pre-IBCLC group (p 5 .021). There was an association with maternal age and continued breast-feeding. Each increase in year of maternal age corresponded to 1.09 greater odds of still providing some breast milk at the 12-month observation window (p 5 .010). Neither term gestation nor previous childbirth was predictive of providing any breast milk at 12 months.

Although all mothers in the IBCLC-A group had access to the expertise of the lactation consultant, not all mothers used the services. Mothers who had access to an IBCLC but did not personally interact with her were still 3.18 times more likely to be providing breast milk at 12 months than mothers in the pre-IBCLC group (p 5 .009). Refer to Table 6 for a more in-depth analysis.

Table 3. Exclusive Feeding of Breast Milk (Multinomial Logistic Regression)

Supplemented With Formula Prior to 1-Month Visit[a]	B	SE B	Wald χ^2	p Value	OR	OR CI
Group[b]	.559	.312	3.230	.073	1.750	0.950–3.222
History of children[c]	−.007	.321	0.001	.982	0.993	0.529–1.862
Term status[d]	.144	.437	0.108	.742	1.155	0.491–2.717
Maternal age	−.033	.032	1.087	.297	0.968	0.910–1.029
Exclusively Breastfed for 1–2 Months						
Group	.602	.344	3.066	.080	1.826	0.931–3.584
History of children	−.371	.361	1.058	.304	0.690	0.340–1.399
Term status	.070	.491	0.020	.887	1.072	0.410–2.804
Maternal age	−.063	.036	3.096	.079	0.939	0.876–1.007

[a]Four+ month breastfeeding category serves as reference category.
[b]Odds ratio displayed calculated for pre-IBCLC group.
[c]Odds ratio displayed calculated for first birth mothers.
[d]Odds ratio displayed calculated for 34–37 weeks gestation (late preterm).

Table 4. Duration of Any Breastfeeding

Group	Infants Fed Any Breast Milk at Initial Visit	Infants Reported to Be Fed Any Breast Milk at Specified Well-Child Visit Interval					
		1-Month Visit	2-Month Visit	4-Month Visit	6-Month Visit	9-Month Visit	12-Month Visit
Pre-IBCLC	120	79.2% (95)	63.3% (76)	50.8% (61)	40.8% (49)	30.0% (36)	14.2% (17)
IBCLC-A	136	79.4% (108)	66.2% (90)	51.5% (70)	45.6% (62)	39.0% (53)	26.5% (36)

Note. IBCLC = International Board Certified Lactation Consultant; IBCLC-A = International Board Certified Lactation Consultant available group.

There were 31 infants in the IBCLC-A group who were receiving both breast milk and formula at the 1-month visit. By the 2-month visit, 8 of these infants had transitioned to exclusively receiving breast milk. In the pre-IBCLC group, none of the 45 infants who were receiving both breast milk and formula at the 1-month visit ever transitioned to exclusive breast milk.

Discussion

This study demonstrated that the presence of an IBCLC in the outpatient setting appears to have a significant positive impact on breastfeeding. Mothers who had access to an IBCLC in the pediatric primary care setting had greater odds of breast-feeding for a longer duration and tended to breastfeed more exclusively than women who did not have such access. Mothers in the IBCLC-A group who did not personally interact with the consultant still proved to be much more likely to meet the American Academy of Pediatrics' (AAP) recommendations to breastfeed for at least 12 months. Although neither gestational age nor a history of having other children increased the odds of exclusive breastfeeding or the duration of breastfeeding, greater maternal age was associated with increased odds a mother would be providing breast milk at the 1-year mark.

In this study, many mothers found the need to supplement with nonhuman milk during the first month of life. This was evident in both of the groups. However, more mothers in the pre-IBCLC had ceased exclusive breastfeeding at each observation window than mothers who had access to an IBCLC.

Of the mothers who were supplementing at the 1-month visit, a quarter of those who had access to the care and guidance of an IBCLC in the primary care setting were able to transition back to exclusive breastfeeding by the second month. This phenomenon did not occur at all in the pre-IBCLC group. Because of the study design, this return to exclusive breastfeeding was not reflected in the numbers of mothers exclusively breastfeeding.

Interestingly, the same percentage of mothers in both the pre-IBCLC group and IBCLC-A group quit breastfeeding prior to the 1-month well-child visit. However, at all the remaining observation windows, more mothers quit breastfeeding at every interval in the pre-IBCLC group than the IBCLC-A group. At the 1-year mark, only the group that had access to an IBCLC met the national recommendations, and far exceeded Pennsylvania's average 1-year breastfeeding rates.

Most infants in both groups were delivered at the same local hospital. Although this facility is not designated as baby-friendly, early postpartum breastfeeding support was available from the same two IBCLCs for both groups. There were no significant changes to birth practices at this birthing facility during the time frames of this study. Other potential confounding factors such as mothers in the pre-IBCLC group seeking assistance from an IBCLC, the level of support mothers derived from internet resources and support groups, or the percentage of mothers who returned to work in each group were not able to be controlled for because of the design of the study as a retrospective chart review.

Table 5. Feeding Any Breast Milk for at Least 1 Year (Binary Logistic Regression)

	B	SE B	Wald χ^2	p Value	OR	OR CI
Group[a]	0.764	.331	5.330	.021	2.147	1.122–4.016
History of children[b]	0.153	.330	0.215	.643	1.165	0.611–2.222
Term status[c]	0.057	.449	0.016	.898	1.059	0.439–2.553
Maternal age	−4.497	.033	6.723	.010	1.090	1.021–1.164

[a]Odds ratio displayed calculated for International Board Certified Lactation Consultant available group (IBCLC-A group).
[b]Odds ratio displayed calculated for first birth mothers.
[c]Odds ratio displayed calculated for term deliveries.

Table 6. Nonconsultant Users—Any Feeding of Breast Milk at 1 Year (Binary Logistic Regression)

	B	SE B	Wald χ^2	p Value	OR	OR CI
Group[a]	1.156	0.440	6.915	0.009	3.178	1.342–7.525
History of children[b]	0.173	0.461	0.141	0.708	1.189	0.482–2.933
Term status[c]	0.079	0.621	0.016	0.898	1.082	0.321–3.654
Maternal age	0.057	0.048	1.400	0.237	1.058	0.963–1.162

[a]Odds ratio displayed calculated for International Board Certified Lactation Consultant available group (IBCLC-A group).
[b]Odds ratio displayed calculated for first birth mothers.
[c]Odds ratio displayed calculated for late preterm deliveries.

An unexpected finding was that women in the IBCLC-A group who did not personally interact with the IBCLC were still significantly more likely to be breastfeeding at 1 year of age as compared to the preIBCLC group. A possible explanation may be that physicians who use an IBCLC are more likely to adhere to AAP recommendations for breastfeeding. Another plausible rationale is that the presence of the IBCLC in the primary care setting promotes conversations and education to healthcare providers regarding the most current breastfeeding knowledge and treatment recommendations. In addition, mothers who are more committed to breastfeeding may seek out a primary care setting that includes the expertise of an IBCLC in their healthcare team.

Implications for Practice and Further Research

This research supports the integration of IBCLCs into the pediatric primary care setting. The presence of an IBCLC in this setting significantly increased the odds of mothers meeting medical recommendations to breastfeed for at least 1 year, and women tended to breastfeed more exclusively for the first 6 months. Further studies are needed to investigate what types of problems mothers encounter in the outpatients setting which prompt them to seek advice from an IBCLC. Information is needed to correlate breastfeeding diagnoses with the intensity and types of interventions implemented by the IBCLC to improve/maintain the integrity of the breastfeeding relationship.

Additional research is needed which differentiates between breastfeeding and providing expressed breast milk. Mothers who are unable to resolve nipple and latch problems often resort to pumping to provide breast milk. Many mothers who are exclusively pumping will quit earlier than they had intended because of the effort of expressing breast milk (Odom et al., 2013).

Not differentiating between feeding at the breast and mothers who were exclusively pumping may have artificially inflated perceptions of breastfeeding success in the first few months, especially in the pre-IBCLC group.

Limitations

This study was conducted in a single pediatric practice that employed one IBCLC. The practice was located in a suburban area, with a homogenous, higher-than-average income patient population. Replication of this study in urban and more diverse populations will produce results that are more generalizable. In addition, breastfeeding duration and exclusivity were based on set windows of observation.

Missing data was a limitation in this study when investigating breastfeeding duration and exclusivity. To eliminate the creation of a potential bias, data sets that were missing study variables were eliminated from further analysis. The elimination of these data sets may have impacted the results.

Conclusions

Mothers who had access to the expertise of an IBCLC were significantly more likely to overcome obstacles and continue breastfeeding. The integration of an IBCLC into the pediatric primary care setting appears to be a viable option to increase breastfeeding exclusivity and duration rates. Enabling mothers to reach breastfeeding goals will have a significant positive impact on the lifelong health of our nation. Affording all mothers access to the expertise of an IBCLC should be a priority action to assist this country in achieving the Healthy People 2020 goals.

References

Bonuck, K., Trombley, B., Freeman, K., & McKee, D. (2005). Randomized controlled trial of a prenatal and postnatal lactation consultant intervention on duration and intensity of breastfeeding up to 12 months. *Pediatrics, 116*(6), 1413–1426. http://dx.doi.org/10.1542/peds.2005-0435

Castrucci, B., Hoover, K., Lim, S., & Maus, K. (2007). Availability of lactation counseling services influences breastfeeding among infants admitted to neonatal intensive care units. *American Journal of Health Promotion, 21*(5), 410–415.

Centers for Disease Control and Prevention. (2012). *Breastfeeding report card 2012, United States: Outcome indicators.* Retrieved from http://www.cdc.gov/breastfeeding/data/reportcard2.htm

Dodgson, J., & Tarrant, M. (2007). Outcomes of a breastfeeding educational intervention for baccalaureate nursing students. *Nurse Education Today, 27*(8), 856–867. http://dx.doi.org/10.1016/j.nedt.2006.12.001

Francis-Clegg, S., & Francis, D. (2011). Improving the "bottomline": Financial justification for the hospital-based lactation consultant role. *Clinical Lactation, 2*(1), 19–25.

Gutowski, J., Walker, M., & Chetwynd, E. (2012). Containing health care costs help in plain sight. *International Board Certified Lactation Consultants: Allied Healthcare Providers Contribute to the Solution* (2nd ed.). Morrisville, NC: United States Lactation Consultant Association.

Hamlyn, B., Brooker, S., Oleinikova, K., & Wands, S. (2002). Infant feeding 2000. *A survey conducted on behalf of the Department of Health, the Scottish Executive, the National Assembly for Wales and the Department of Health, Social Services and Public Safety in Northern Ireland.* London, United Kingdom: The Stationery Office.

Lewallen, L., Dick, M., Flowers, J., Powell, W., Zickefoose, K., Wall, Y., & Price, Z. (2006). Breastfeeding support and early cessation. *Journal of Obstetric, Gynecologic, and Neonatal Nursing, 35*(2), 166–172.

Mannel, R., & Mannel, R. S. (2006). Staffing for hospital lactation programs: Recommendations from a tertiary care teaching hospital. *Journal of Human Lactation, 22*(409), 409–417. http://dx.doi.org/10.1177/0890334406294166

McDowell, M., Wang, C., & Kennedy-Stephenson, J. (2008). *Breastfeeding in the United States: Findings from the National Health and Nutrition Examination Surveys 1999–2006* (NCHS data briefs, no. 5). Hyattsville, MD: National Center for Health Statistics.

Moore, E., & Coty, M. (2006). Prenatal and postpartum focus groups with primiparas: Breastfeeding attitudes, support, barriers, self-efficacy, and intention. *Journal of Pediatric Health Care, 20*(1), 35–46. http://dx.doi.org/10.1016/j .pedhc.2005.08.007

Noel-Weiss, J., Boersma, S., & Kujawa-Myles, S. (2012). Questioning current definitions for breastfeeding research. *International Breastfeeding Journal, 7*(1), 9. http://dx.doi.org/10.1186/ 1746-4358-7-9

Odom, E., Li, R., Scanlon, K., Perrine, C., & GrummerStrawn, L, (2013). Reasons for earlier than desired cessation of breastfeeding. *Pediatrics, 131*(3), e726–e732. Retrieved from http://pediatrics. aappublications.org/content/ early/2013/02/13/peds.2012-1295

Osband, Y., Altman, R., Patrick, P., & Edwards, K. (2011). Breastfeeding education and support services offered to pediatric residents in the U.S. *Academic Pediatrics, 11*(1), 75–77. http://dx.doi.org/10.1016/j.acap.2010.11.002

Ryan, A., Wenjun, Z., & Acosta, A. (2002). Breastfeeding continues to increase into the new millennium. *Pediatrics, 110*(6), 1103–1109.

Thurman, S., & Allen, P. (2008). Integrating lactation consultants into primary health care services: Are lactation consultants affecting breastfeeding success? *Pediatric Nursing, 34*(5), 419–425.

United States Department of Health and Human Services. (2011). *Surgeon general's call to action to support breastfeeding.* Washington, DC: United States Department of Health and Human Services, Office of the Surgeon General.

Wagner, E., Chantry, C., Dewey, K., & Nommsen-Rivers, L. (2013). Breastfeeding concerns at 3 and 7 days postpartum and feeding status at 2 months. *Pediatrics, 132*(4), 865–875. http://dx.doi. org/10:1542/peds.2013-0724

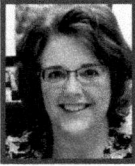

Cynthia A. Morris, DNP, RN, IBCLC, RLC, has been assisting mothers and babies with breastfeeding in the acute care setting since 1991. She became an International Board Certified Lactation Consultant in 2005 and recently earned her doctorate of nursing practice. She is employed as an assistant professor at Westmoreland County Community College where she instructs prelicensure nursing students. She continues her commitment to breastfeeding by working as a lactation consultant in the acute care setting. She resides and works in Southwestern Pennsylvania.

Judith I. Gutowski, BA, IBCLC, RLC, has a BA in psychology and has worked in the field of lactation as a La Leche League Leader and an International Board Certified Lactation Consultant since 1995. She is employed in a pediatric practice. Judy is a legislative and policy advocate for the U.S. Lactation Consultant Association striving to improve access to lactation care provided by International Board Certified Lactation Consultants.

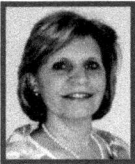

USLCA

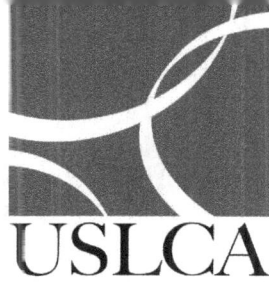

Hospitalization for Nipple Confusion
A Method to Restore Healthy Breastfeeding

Asti Praborini, MD, IBCLC | Hani Purnamasari, MD

Agusnawati Munandar, MD, IBCLC, CIMI

Ratih Ayu Wulandari, MD, IBCLC

Keywords: nipple confusion, tongue-tie, bottle-feeding, breastfeeding, relactation, initiation of lactation

Background: *The World Health Organization has encouraged all facilities providing maternity services and care for newborn infants to adopt the "10 steps" of successful breastfeeding. This includes not giving artificial teats to breastfeeding infants because they may cause nipple confusion. We present a multimodal hospitalization protocol for infants with nipple confusion, a multimodal relactation method that supports breastfeeding couplets.*

Purpose: *To investigate the effectiveness of hospitalization as an intervention for nipple confusion.*

Method: *Data related to nipple confusion in patients hospitalized between January and December 2012 at Kemang*

Medical Care, Jakarta, Indonesia, was reviewed. Survival analysis was performed to evaluate the relationship between infant age and intervention outcomes.

Results: *There were 58 cases of nipple confusion during the study period. Most subjects (96.6%) totally rejected breast contact. Forty-six cases (79.3%) used bottles because of tongue-tie. The length of hospitalization varied from 1 (56.9%) to 5 days (3.4%). Fifty-three cases (91.4%) were able to successfully breastfeed using our protocol. Younger babies had greater breastfeeding success.*

Conclusion: *Hospitalization for nipple confusion with multi-modal management is effective for treating nipple confusion. Tongue-tie can lead to difficulties in initiating breastfeeding, and early introduction to artificial teats can lead to nipple confusion. Early detection and treatment is desirable.*

Breastfeeding is the most natural way for mother and infant to bond while providing nutrition, warmth, and security. Compared to feeding the baby with formula milk, breastfeeding has numerous health benefits. Many studies have provided strong evidence that breastfeeding reduces a wide range of infectious diseases including bacterial meningitis, bacteremia, diarrhea, respiratory tract infections, otitis media, urinary tract infections, and late-onset sepsis in preterm infants. Breast-feeding also decrease the chances of childhood malignancy and allergic and metabolic diseases, such as asthma, diabetes mellitus, and hypercholesterolemia (Gartner et al., 2005).

Breastfeeding also provides important health benefits to mothers including decreased postpartum bleeding and more rapid uterine involution. These benefits are attributable to increased concentrations of oxytocin, decreased menstrual blood loss, increased child spacing because of lactational amenorrhea, earlier return to prepregnancy weight, a decreased risk of breast and ovarian cancer, and possibly, a decreased risk of hip fractures and osteoporosis in the postmenopausal period (Association of Women's Health, Obstetric and Neonatal Nurses, 2015). Babies who are not breastfed are, therefore, at greater risk of suffering health problems. In addition, a lack of breastfeeding decreases maternal–infant bonding, which is important for neurodevelopment (Liu, Leung, & Yang, 2014).

To support breastfeeding, the World Health Organization (WHO) encourages all facilities providing maternity services and care for newborn infants to follow the "Ten Steps to Successful Breastfeeding" including "give no artificial teats or pacifiers (also called dummies or soothers) to breastfeeding infants" (Vallenas & Savage, 1998, p. 74).

Suckling is a way to feed an infant from the breast; in contrast, sucking is the oral motor activity that transfers milk. It is more difficult to teach an infant to suckle from the breast if he or she is accustomed to feeding from a bottle, even if the breast is producing milk. Infants who are bottle-fed may develop a preference for artificial teats over the breast (Vallenas & Savage, 1998). Babies who exclusively breastfeed are known to develop different sucking patterns compared to babies who are fed by bottle (Moral et al., 2010).

A Japanese study of breastfed and bottle-fed infants shows that suckling (the front to back, wavelike movement) transitions to sucking (a straight up and down movement of the tongue and jaw) in bottle-fed infants because of mechanical differences between breast and artificial nipples and the oral cavity (Genna, 2012). Several studies have analyzed the electrical activity of the masseter muscle during breast- and bottle-feeding of newborn infants using surface electromyography (França, Sousa, Aragão, & Costa, 2014). Together, these results suggest that masseter activity is significantly greater in breastfed than bottle-fed newborns. In contrast to breastfed infants, bottle-fed infants use the buccinator and orbicularis oris muscles more and the mentalis and masseter muscles less (Genna, 2012).

During breastfeeding, the tongue actively brings the nipple into the mouth, shapes the nipple and areola into a teat, and stabilizes the teat's position. This is different to bottle-feeding in which only the tongue is needed to stabilize the nipple's position, and the artificial nipple does not need to be drawn into the mouth (Walker, 2013). Furthermore, these mechanical differences are also reflected in the movement of fluid: During breastfeeding, fluid moves from the high-pressure ducts inside the breast (created by fluid volume and the milk ejection reflex) to an area of low pressure inside the baby's mouth (caused by the suction or vacuum created by sealing the oral cavity and enlarging it when the tongue and jaw drop). During bottle-feeding, either suction or compression determine efficient fluid flow, depending on the type of nipple and its opening (Walker, 2013).

The early introduction of bottles to infants has been shown to result in ineffective suckling and frustration when babies try to breastfeed. As a consequence, breast rejection is a common cause of breastfeeding failure (Newman & Wilmott, 1990). The refusal of a baby to latch after introduction of an artificial nipple or bottle is called nipple confusion, which refers to the infant's difficulty in achieving the correct oral configuration, latching technique, and suckling pattern necessary for successful breastfeeding after bottle-feeding or other exposures to an artificial nipple (Neifert, Lawrence, & Seacat, 1995).

Hospitalization for nipple confusion is sometimes used to support the mother–baby dyad to achieve a healthy breastfeeding relationship. One such program has been implemented in our hospital and has helped many mothers and babies to restore a happy breastfeeding relationship. Our hospital is a mother and children's hospital in Jakarta, Indonesia. The hospital operates a lactation clinic 12 hours daily, which consists of physicians who also act as lactation counselors/consultants divided into three shifts per day. Lactation doctors take a 40-hour breastfeeding counseling course, and courses on lactation management, complimentary feeding for breastfed babies, and kangaroo mother care. The lactation doctor consults patients at lactation clinic and conducts rounds in postnatal care and to see mothers and infants hospitalized because of nipple confusion, mastitis, abscess, or other lactation problems such as nursing strike or adoptive nursing. Here, we aimed to investigate the effectiveness of hospitalization and multimodal management as an intervention for nipple confusion.

Method

Patients, Data Collection, and Diagnosis of Nipple Confusion

Data were collected between January and December 2012. Fifty-eight mothers attended lactation clinic concerned about breast rejection at Kemang Medical Care, a Baby-Friendly hospital located in Jakarta, Indonesia.

A breastfeeding history was taken from participants including questions about when a bottle was introduced. The lactation doctor observed each mother breastfeed her baby and evaluated the mother's breasts, and the baby's mouth, to iden-tify sore nipples, mastitis, breasts abscesses, tongue-tie, and/or lip-tie. Bottle-feeding, or an artificial nipple, were commonly used by mothers and family when faced with breastfeeding difficulties caused by tongue-tie and/or lip-tie, such as nipple pain, long feeding, or a fussy baby.

Nipple confusion was reported if the babies refused the breast, arched, cried, or screamed at the breast, or pushed the breast away (Newman & Wilmott, 1990).

This was considered different to a nursing strike, in which the baby suddenly refuses to nurse after breastfeeding successfully, often because of another problem, such as teething, a stuffy nose, ear infections, a reaction to being left unattended, recent separation of baby from mother, or if the baby has bitten the mother and her response was a loud scream that frightened the baby (Cadwell & Turner-Maffei, 2013).

Tongue-tie was defined by looking at the frenulum's attachment to the tongue using the Coryllos classification: Type 1—the tip of the tongue is in front of the gums; Type 2—2–4 mm behind the tip of the tongue, attached to or slightly behind the gums; Type 3—attached to the middle of the tongue until the floor of the mouth; or Type 4—at the base of the tongue, thick, shiny, and not very elastic (Coryllos, Watson Genna, & Salloum, 2004).

Hospitalization Protocol

If the baby totally refused the breast, we suggested hospitalization of both mother and baby to restore their breastfeeding relationship. Hospitalization for nipple confusion is important to increase patient compliance and provide a supportive environment for mother and baby to reconnect. In Indonesia, most new parents live in a house with their extended family, with grandparents or relatives living in the same house giving poor breastfeeding advice and making it difficult to resolve the problem without hospitalization. In most cases, hospitalization was funded personally, although their insurance companies reimbursed some patients.

In our hospitalization program, mother and baby were roomed for 24 hours, received food and any prescribed medication, were visited by lactation doctor three times a day to help mother breastfeed, and were visited by a pediatrician once a day to reassure the mother that the baby was doing well.

Relactation is a complex process and needs a holistic approach. During hospitalization, mother and baby were reconnected by experiencing 24-hour skin-to-skin contact wrapped in a traditional cloth and covered by a gown with breaks only for mother/baby bath time or prayer (Figure 1).

In the early days of hospitalization, if the baby still refused the breast, milk was offered using alternative methods to a bottle: expressed breast milk, pasteurized donor breast milk, or formula, depending on the parents' preference. A nurse administered milk to the baby via a syringe, glass, or spoon. The amount of the milk offered was only three-quarters of the amount estimated as the baby's daily requirement to allow the baby to experience slight hunger.

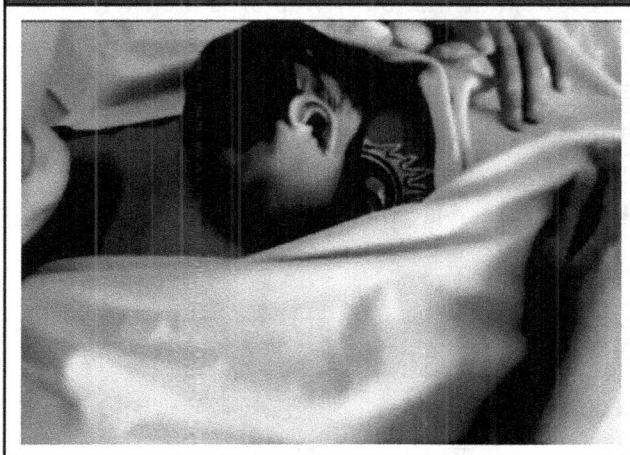

Figure 1. Skin to skin will make mother and baby reconnect.

A baby with nipple confusion can be very angry when offered the breast. Therefore, we administered the antihistamine chlorpheniramine maleate (CPM) to the baby. CPM is an H1 antihistamine that is indicated in perennial and seasonal allergic rhinitis, uncomplicated allergic skin disorders, or as a therapy for anaphylactic reactions. CPM has sedative properties and may impair alertness (Ebadi, 2008). The dose for baby is 0.1 mg/kg 6–8 hours orally, given as a compound medicine. Pharmaceutical compounding is an important part of healthcare and pharmacy practice, and an important practice in many patients who cannot take traditional medication, such as pediatric patients (Riley, 2004). In our experience, the baby was calmer after 1–2 days of CPM and was more likely to take the breast. At this point, CPM was stopped.

When the baby wanted to take the breast, a lactation aid of a 5F gastric tube (40 cm) and a 50-ml syringe taped to the mother's breast and shoulder was used (Figure 2). This lactation aid could be filled with mother's milk, pasteurized donor breast milk, or formula, depending on the mother's stage of Lactogenesis. If nipple confusion occurred during Lactogenesis II (3–8 days after birth), the mother was not given a galactogogue, and the baby was breastfed with a lactation aid filled with the mother's expressed breast milk. However, if confusion occurred during Lactogenesis III (after Day 9), and the mother's milk supply had already decreased, mother was given domperidone therapy and acupuncture with the lactation aid containing pasteurized donor breast milk or formula.

If the baby had upper lip-tie and/or tongue-tie, a pediatrician performed a frenotomy after the baby had exhibited an interest in breastfeeding. In preparation for frenotomy, the baby was swaddled to immobilize the arms and legs and laid supine on the examination table. An assistant helped with the procedure: The frenulum was disinfected with povidone iodine and snipped using blunt-ended sterile scissors and sterile gauze used to attain hemostasis. We favored not using general anesthesia to perform this procedure because this is likely to delay breastfeeding. Frenotomy is an effective, simple, and safe treatment for tongue-tied babies experiencing breast-feeding difficulties. (Praborini, Purnamasari, Munandar, & Wulandari, 2015).

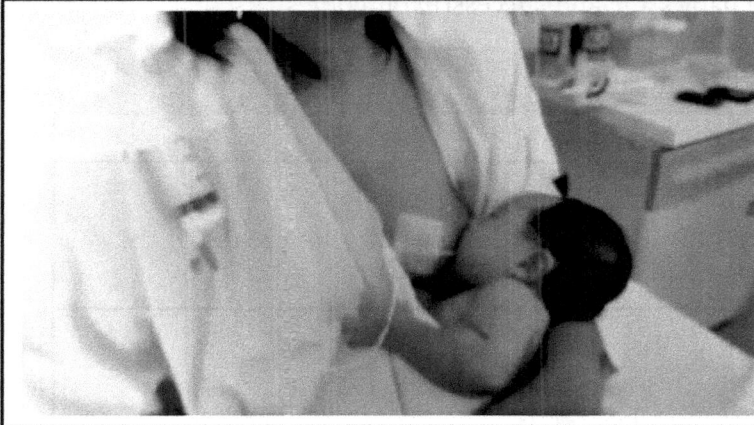

Figure 2. Lactation aid to make baby happy at the breast.

Tongue and lip exercises post-frenotomy are important to reduce frenulum scarring, and the tongue must be mobilized immediately by exercises several times daily (Olivi, Signore, Olivi, & Genovese, 2012). Babies with oral dysfunction because of tongue-tie and nipple confusion will need to learn skills before they can feed properly from their mother's breast, which can be facilitated with oral motor exercises (Sanches, 2004). In our protocol, we taught the mother to gently massage their baby's upper lip, lower lip, and cheeks, and how to pull the upper lip outwards, gently touch the tongue downward, and touch the palate, buccal area, and gum to stimulate tongue movements to all areas inside the mouth and stretch the post-frenotomy site. These maneuvers were performed five times daily for 3 weeks.

"Success" was defined as when baby breastfed effectively at the breast for 15 minutes with or without supplemental aids. If a baby refused the breast or breastfed ineffectively and/or the parents went home, this was defined as "not success."

Survival analysis (SPSS Version 19, IBM Statistics, Chicago, Illinois) was performed to evaluate the relationship between the baby's age and successful outcomes.

Table 1. Subject Characteristics	
Characteristics	N (%)
Sex	
Boy	38 (65,5)
Girl	20 (34,5)
Age	
0–30 days	16 (27,6)
1–3 months	25 (43,1)
4–6 months	15 (25,9)
>6 months	2 (3,4)
Place of birth	
KMC	6 (10,3)
Outside KMC	52 (89,7)
Latching	
With tongue-tie	46 (79,3)
Without tongue-tie	12 (20,7)

Results

Fifty-eight cases of nipple confusion were hospitalized during the study period, 52 of which were born outside Kemang Medical Care Hospital. The subject characteristics are detailed in Table 1. Forty-one cases had (70.7%) received breast milk substitute by bottle, 15 cases (25.9%) received breast milk by bottle, 1 case (1.7%) only latched to the breast with a nipple shield, and 1 case (1.7%) only wanted to drink from a glass.

Twenty-nine cases (50%) had received breast milk substitute by bottle in the hospital, 13 cases (22.4%) were given bottles at home, and 47 cases (81%) were fed by bottle within 1 week of birth. Fifty-six (96.6%) babies totally refused the breast. Most babies (46 cases, 76.3%) had difficulty in latching on to the nipple because of tongue-tie. Two cases (3.4%) had difficulty in latching on after a frenotomy and received expressed breast milk with a bottle. Most cases (53 cases, 91.4%) were deemed "successful" after hospitalization and babies were able to breastfeed; the others discharged from hospital before breastfeeding was well established because the parents chose to leave. The length of hospitalization varied from less than 24 hours (one case, 1.7%) to 5 days (two cases, 3.4%), as shown in Figure 3. Survival analysis showed that the younger the age of a baby at hospitalization, the higher the success in getting the baby to breastfeed (Figure 4).

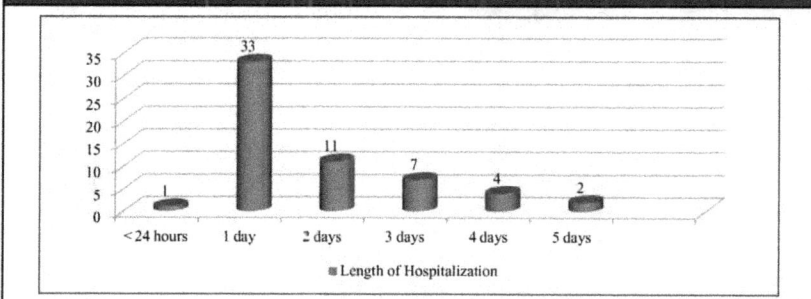

Figure 3. Number of cases and length of hospitalization.

Discussion

The WHO encourages all facilities providing maternity services and care for newborn infants to adopt the "10 steps," which includes not giving artificial teats to breastfeeding infants because they are known to contribute to nipple confusion. However, not all hospitals are "babyfriendly." In our study, 29 babies (50%) received formula while in the hospital in the neonatal period, and 47 cases (81%) received bottles within 1 week of birth. This large number identifies a lack of breastfeeding support early in babies' lives in some institutions. Difficulty in latching on because of tongue-tie was the primary reason for bottle-feeding (46 cases, 76.3%).

Figure 4. Success rate of the hospitalization protocol with respect to the baby's age. The younger the age, the higher the success rate of returning the baby to the breast.

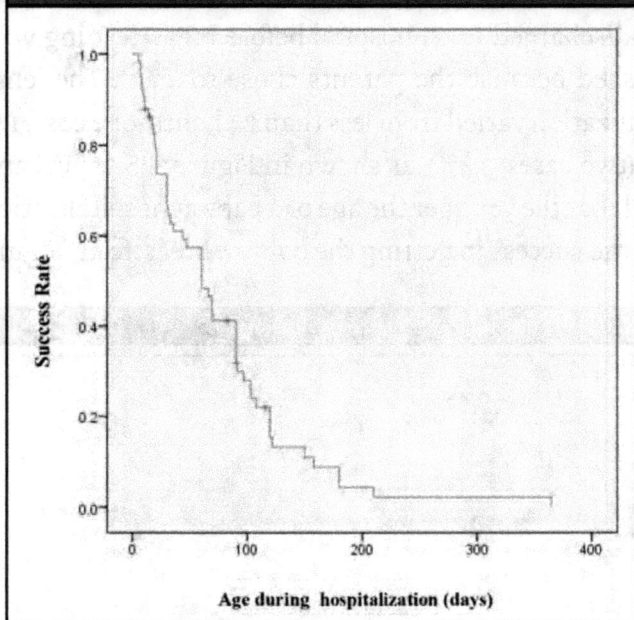

Sucking from the breast and from artificial teats are different processes. Not all babies can suck from both breast and teats, or are able to easily switch from breast to bottle or bottle to breast. Nipple confusion occurs via various different mechanisms related to the breast and bottle. In our study, bottle-feeding resulted in 56 babies totally refusing the breast (96.6%), whereas 1 baby (1.7%) would only latch with a nipple shield in place, and 1 baby (1.7%) only wanted to drink with a glass.

Cultural and psychological factors also contribute to nipple confusion. On our study, some people believed that the baby was crying because of hunger and that the breast could not provide sufficient food but a bottle could: 13 cases (22.4%) received bottles at home. In Indonesia, new parents usually stay with their extended family so that the grandmother can help with babysitting. In our experience, parents usually receive poor breastfeeding advice from the extended family.

Hospitalization for nipple confusion provided a positive environment for both mother and baby. Full support from counselors and nurses helped mothers' confidence in breastfeeding their babies. Skin-to-skin contact for 24 hours reintroduced the baby to the mother. Tactile and verbal contact is optimal during skin-to-skin contact and makes it easier for the baby to return to the breast. A Cochrane systemic review has shown that early skin-to-skin contact over long periods contributes to a positive effect that promotes exclusive breast-feeding (Mahmood, Jamal, & Khan, 2011). Skin-to-skin contact during breastfeeding enhances positive maternal feelings and shortens the time it takes to resolve severe latch-on problems in infants (Svensson, Velandia, Matthiesen, Welles-Nyström, & Widström, 2013). This results in mother and baby being more comfortable and happy, and leads to better bonding. If the baby still refused the breast during the early days of hospitalization, we used a cup as a transition from bottle to breast because masseter activity during cup feeding is similar to that seen in breastfeeding (França et al., 2014). For babies who only wanted a cup, we used a syringe filled with milk to give to the baby. After the baby wanted to take the breast, frenotomy should be performed in babies with tongue-tie and/or lip-tie to correct the baby's sucking skills, followed by lactation aids to help the baby become comfortable at the breast. A bottle-fed baby will be happy with lactation aids because it mimics the fast flow of the bottle and delivers milk without much effort from the baby (Lauwers & Swisher, 2010). Therefore, the purpose of the lactation aid is to increase the flow of milk so that the infant obtains milk from the nipple, and the lactation aid on each suck of the breast.

The purpose of relactation is to reintroduce the baby to the breast so that the baby can receive adequate nutrition from the breast; thus, the mother should have sufficient milk supply. If nipple confusion occurs during Lactogenesis II (3–8 days after birth), the mother was not given a galactogogue because of insufficient milk supply.

Lactation aids filled with mother's expressed breast milk should be taped to the breast to mimic the fast flow of the bottle and can be removed after the baby starts to suckle effectively from the breast. However, if nipple confusion occurs during Lactogenesis III (after Day 9), the mother's milk supply has usually decreased because of low demand. The mother should therefore be given domperidone and acupuncture together with a lactation aid containing pasteurized donor breast milk or formula. At this stage, one can also consider using supplemental nursing systems to help the baby to gain weight. Lactation aids can be removed after the mother has sufficient milk supply, which usually occurs after a relatively long period of time. Domperidone is a dopamine D2 receptor antagonist that increases milk volume rapidly within 48 hours. At a therapeutic dose of 3 3 10 mg to 3 3 30 mg/day, side effects include weight gain (11.7%), headache (9.8%), cardiac arrhythmias (0.8%), and depression (0.9%). Over the course of treatment, mothers need to slowly taper off the dose to avoid withdrawal effects (Ruddock, 2005). However, domperidone is safe for the infant (Hale & Rowe, 2004).

We also showed that the younger the baby, the higher the success rate of returning the baby to the breast. Hospitalization for nipple confusion had an overall success rate of 91.4% and was, therefore, a highly effective method that can contribute to a successful breastfeeding couplet.

Our study was difficult to compare to other studies because to the best of our knowledge, only one similar study has been reported (Newman & Wilmott, 1990). Furthermore, our study was relatively small in size and retrospective. A prospective multicenter study is needed to fully evaluate the effectiveness of our method in a larger population.

Conclusion

Tongue-tie may interrupt or prevent optimal latching to the breast during a baby's first day of life, and introduction of an artificial nipple may cause nipple confusion and interrupt exclusive breastfeeding. Early detection and treatment of tongue-tie and nipple confusion is very important to achieve successful breastfeeding. Hospitalization and a multimodal approach to the management of nipple confusion is effective and can contribute to a successful breastfeeding and should be implemented as quickly as possible because younger infants appear to have better outcomes.

References

Association of Women's Health, Obstetric and Neonatal Nurses. (2015). *Breastfeeding. Journal of Obstetric, Gynecologic, & Neonatal Nursing, 44*(1), 145–150. http://dx.doi.org/10.1111/1552-6909.12530

Cadwell, K., & Turner-Maffei, C. (2013). *Breastfeeding A-Z*. Burlington, MA: Jones & Bartlett.

Coryllos, E., Watson Genna, C., & Salloum, A. (2004, Summer). Congenital tongue-tie and its impact on breast feeding. *American Academy of Pediatrics Section on Breastfeeding Newsletter*, 1–6.

Ebadi, M. S. (2008). *Desk reference of clinical pharmacology*. Boca Raton, FL: CRC Press.

França, E. C. L., Sousa, C. B., Aragão, L. C., & Costa, L. R. (2014). Electromyographic analysis of masseter muscle in newborns during suction in breast, bottle, or cup feeding. *BMC Pregnancy and Childbirth, 14*, 154. http://dx.doi.org/10.1186/1471-2393-14-154

Gartner, L. M., Morton, J., Lawrence, R. A, Naylor, A. J., O'Hare, D., Schanler, R. J., & Eidelman, A. I. (2005). Breastfeeding and the use of human milk. *Pediatrics, 115*(2), 496–506. http://dx.doi.org/10.1542/peds.2004-2491

Genna, C. W. (2012). Supporting sucking skills in breastfeeding infants. Sudbury, MA: Jones & Bartlett. Hale, T. W., & Rowe, H. E. (2004). Medications and mothers' milk. Amarillo, TX: Pharmasoft Medical.

Lauwers, J., & Swisher, A. (2010). *Counseling the nursing mother*. Sudbury, MA: Jones & Bartlett.

Liu, J., Leung, P., & Yang, A. (2014). Breastfeeding and active bonding protects against children's internalizing behavior problems. *Nutrients, 6*(1), 76–89. http://dx.doi.org/10.3390/nu6010076

Mahmood, I., Jamal, M., & Khan, N. (2011). Effect of motherinfant early skin-to-skin contact on breastfeeding status: A randomized controlled trial. *Journal of the College of Physicians and Surgeons—Pakistan, 21*(10), 601–605.

Moral, A., Bolibar, I., Seguranyes, G., Ustrell, J. M., Sebastiá, G., Martínez-Barba, C., & Ríos, J. (2010). *Mechanics of sucking: Comparison between bottle feeding and breastfeeding*. BMC Pediatrics, 10, 6. http://dx.doi.org/10.1186/1471-2431-10-6

Neifert, M., Lawrence, R., & Seacat, J. (1995). Nipple confusion: Toward a formal definition. *The Journal of Pediatrics, 126*(6), S125–S129.

Newman, J., & Wilmott, B. (1990). *Breast rejection: A little-appreciated cause of lactation failure. Canadian Family Physician, 36*, 449–453.

Olivi, G., Signore, A., Olivi, M., & Genovese, M. D. (2012). Lingual frenectomy: Functional evaluation and new therapeutical approach. *European Journal of Paediatric Dentistry, 13*(2), 101–106. Retrieved from http://www.ncbi.nlm.nih.gov/pubmed/22762170

Praborini, A., Purnamasari, H., Munandar, A., & Wulandari, R. A. (2015). Early frenotomy improves breastfeeding outcomes for tongue-tied infants. *Clinical Lactation, 6*(1), 9–15. http://dx.doi.org/10.1891/2158-0782.6.1.9

Riley, R. (2004). *The regulation of pharmaceutical compounding and the determination of need: Balancing access and autonomy with patient safety.* Harvard Law School, Cambridge, MA.

Ruddock, B. (2005). Domperidone and lactation. *Canadian Pharmacists Journal, 138*(2), 28–29.

Sanches, M. T. C. (2004). Clinical management of oral disorders in breastfeeding. *Jornal de Pediatria, 80*(Suppl. 5), S155–S162. http://dx.doi.org/10.1590/S0021-75572004000700007

Svensson, K. E., Velandia, M. I., Matthiesen, A. S. T., WellesNyström, B. L., & Widström, A. M. E. (2013). Effects of mother-infant skin-to-skin contact on severe latch-on problems in older infants: A randomized trial. *International Breastfeeding Journal, 8*(1), 1. http://dx.doi.org/10.1186/1746-4358-8-1

Vallenas, C., & Savage, F. (1998). Evidence for the ten steps to successful breastfeeding. *Geneva, Switzerland: WHO Child Health and Development Unit, 1997.*

Walker, M. (2013). *Breastfeeding management for the clinician.* Sudbury, MA: Jones & Bartlett

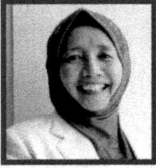

Asti Praborini, MD, IBCLC, is a granny of a successful breastfeeding mother. Having 26 years of experience as pediatrician convinced her that nothing is more valuable than breastfeeding, for both mother and baby. As a national speaker, she campaigns the benefit of breastfeeding despite the loads of breast milk substitute marketing. She built the first dreamed hospital-based lactation team in Indonesia that works ultimately to help mother breastfeed her baby. She is practicing frenotomy for anterior as well as posterior tonguetie and lip-tie, established her method for hospitalization of nipple confusion, supplementation, adoptive nursing, and many others. She also devoted her time to give pro bono services to the poor in pediatric clinic of Layanan Kesehatan Cuma-Cuma (LKC) Dompet Dhuafa and received LKC award in 2011. She is now the chairwoman of the Indonesian International Lactation Consultant Association.

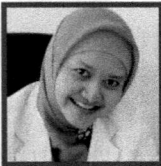

Hani Purnamasari, MD, is a pediatrician who devoted her time in the lactation field after she found many babies were having excessive weight loss and failure to thrive because of breastfeeding difficulties. She is joining the lactation team and now helping many mothers to achieve their breastfeeding goals. She is practicing frenotomy for anterior as well as posterior tongue-tie and lip-tie. Dr. Hani often speaks to promote the benefit of breastfeeding, and her best experience was sharing the same stage with Dr. Jack Newman (pediatrician) at the Seminar and Workshop of Breastfeeding Update on Daily Practice in Jakarta, Indonesia.

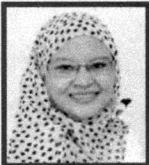

Agusnawati Munandar, MD, IBCLC, CIMI, is a successful breastfeeding mother of two. She is working in a lactation clinic of baby-friendly hospitals and earned her IBCLC degree in 2013. She is involved in lactation teams, which help many mothers to achieve their breastfeeding goals such as practicing frenotomy for anterioras well as posterior tongue-tie and lip-tie, hospitalization for nipple confusion, supplementation, adoptive nursing, and others.

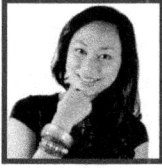

Ratih Ayu Wulandari, MD, IBCLC, entered the lactation field once she realized that breastfeeding mothers need help and support. Having experienced breastfeeding her tongue-tie baby made her support early frenotomy. She is now joining the lactation team and practicing frenotomy for anterior as well as posterior tongue-tie and lip-tie. She believes attachment parenting is the best way to nurture a child and shares the thought on her blog www.menjadiibu.com.

USLCA

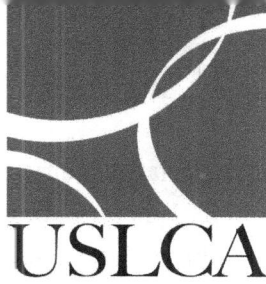

Improving Maternity Practices and Working Toward Baby-Friendly in Hangzhou, China

Kathleen Kendall-Tackett, PhD, IBCLC, RLC, FAPA

Keywords: breastfeeding, postpartum depression, Hangzhou

Hangzhou is a city of 21 million on the coast of Eastern China. The Hangzhou AIMA Maternity Hospital invited me to spend a week training staff and teaching new parents about depression and breastfeeding. This is a private maternity hospital that serves both international and Chinese clientele. Many of the parents had basic questions about labor, breastfeeding, and postpartum. This article describes some of the programs the hospital put into place to increase breastfeeding, lower their cesarean section rate, and now, address postpartum depression.

In May 2015, I was invited to spend a week at the Hangzhou AIMA Maternity Hospital in Hangzhou, China. Hangzhou is the capital of the Zhejiang Province in Eastern China. It is on the coast between Shanghai and Ningbo. I was invited to train their staff about postpartum depression and breastfeeding. I did two training sessions for the hospital staff and six pre- and postnatal classes for parents.

Hangzhou is the fourth largest city in China, with a population of 21 million people. It is a major tourist attraction for the Chinese and is an affluent city. Even in the middle of the week, the tourist sites were packed with people. It is also a very mobile-friendly society, and most of the young people walked around carrying their phones in their hands. Facebook, Google, and other social networking sites are blocked in China. But there are Chinese equivalents and many young Chinese spend their time on a social site called "We Text."

There are very few Westerners in Hangzhou, and the ones I saw at the tourist sites were speaking German. I was often the only Westerner and was enough of an oddity that people would openly stare. I would smile at them, and they would usually respond with friendly grins and waves. (And a few people gestured that they wanted to take a picture with me.)

This hospital is Chinese but was founded by Americans. They are a private maternity hospital and have a large clientele among the internationals who live in Hangzhou. They also have many Chinese patients who have private health insurance. Some spoke a bit of English, but most did not. The hospital furnished me with a wonderful translator, Alisa Hu, who spent the week with me. I'm so glad they gave me a translator because it would have been tough to get around without her. There are English words on signs, but they are often not very helpful. For example, the local convenience store was called "You Easy."

The younger people had a wonderful sense of style, and they were very curious about Westerners. A couple of young women I met told my translator that they could never tell the age of White women. I laughed and said that we often said the same thing about Asian women. They also asked me a lot of questions about hair. Did Westerners color their hair? Yes. Did they have perms? Also yes. Chinese women are also starting to perm and color their hair. On my first night, we went to a high-end shopping mall for dinner. Alisa asked me if I normally shopped at these stores. I taught her the word outlet.

At the Hospital

The AIMA Maternity Hospital was taking several steps to change both their birth and breastfeeding practices (Figure 1). They have started a doula program, have midwives, and they are fairly far along in their work toward Baby-Friendly. They have a large sign in their courtyard listing the 10 steps (Figure 2) and have another large sign in their teaching room announcing their launch of their Baby-Friendly initiative that they had their staff sign (Figure 3). They are working to lower their cesarean section rate, which is currently more than 40%. They also want to improve their breastfeeding rate. As you can see from the sign that was posted in the Shanghai airport (Figure 4), they still live in a culture where bottle feeding is the norm. They want to change that for their patients.

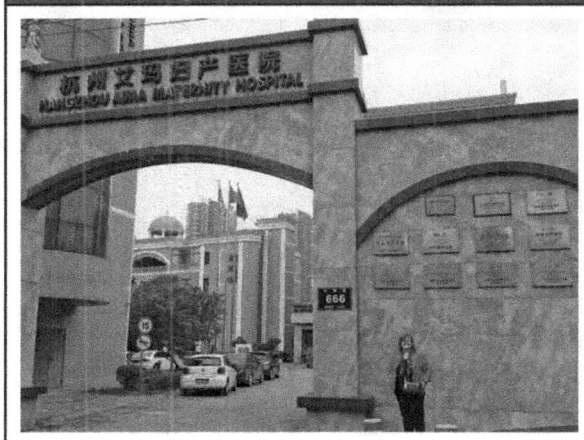

Figure 1. Out in front of the Hangzhou AIMA Maternity Hospital.

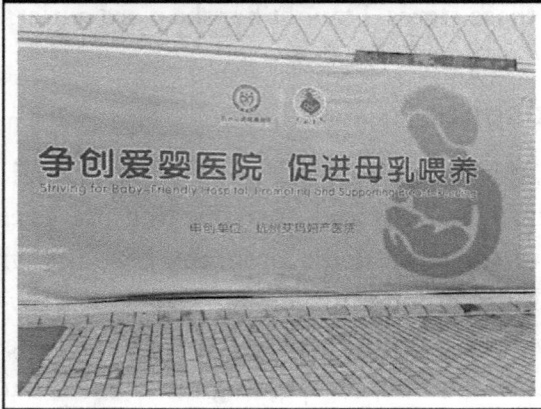

Figure 2. Huge sign in the hospital courtyard listing the 10 steps.

One thing that surprised me was that all of their breastfeeding materials had White women on them (see Figure 3). I was curious and asked them about it. I wondered why they didn't have Chinese women on their materials. They said that they were trying to appeal to their international clientele and no one seemed to think anything of it.

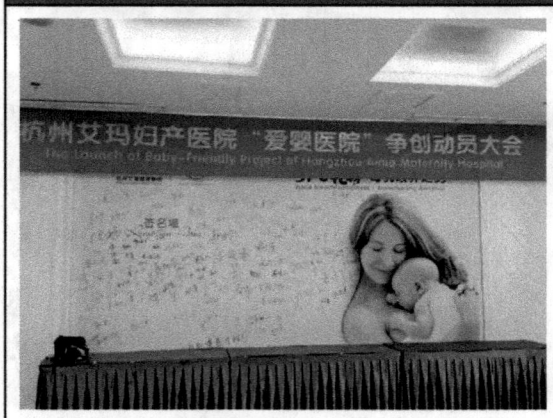

Figure 3. Sign in education room announcing the launch of Baby-Friendly Project.

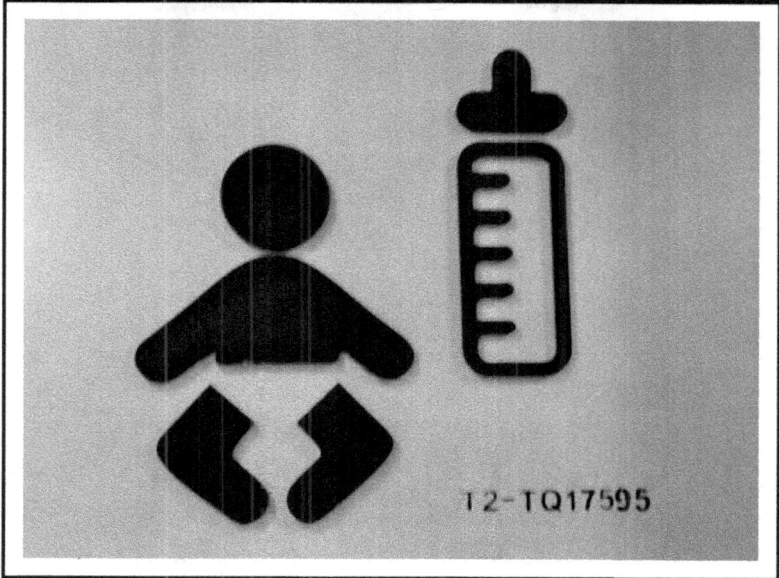

Figure 4. Bottle-feeding symbol outside women's restroom in Shanghai.

Staff Trainings

I taught two trainings on depression and breastfeeding for the nurses and medical staff. While teaching these, I met a lovely midwife named Liz Jiang (Figure 5). She told me it was her dream to become an IBCLC. I sent a quick email to Cathy Carothers (once I figured out how to bypass the block on Google). Cathy sent me the name of an IBCLC in Shanghai. Liz is now connected with a group of IBCLCs in China. She is thrilled. She recently wrote to me to tell me that she attended an 8-day training course in Shanghai for aspiring IBCLCs (Figure 6). She is well on her way.

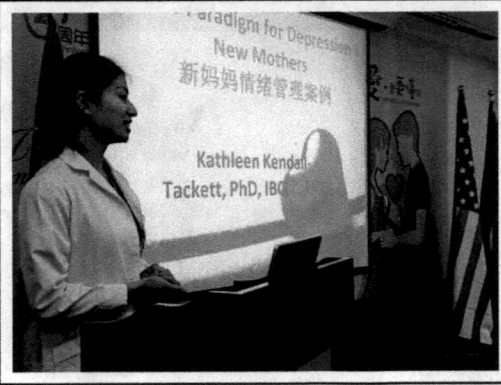

Figure 5. Teaching a staff training with midwife Liz Jiang.

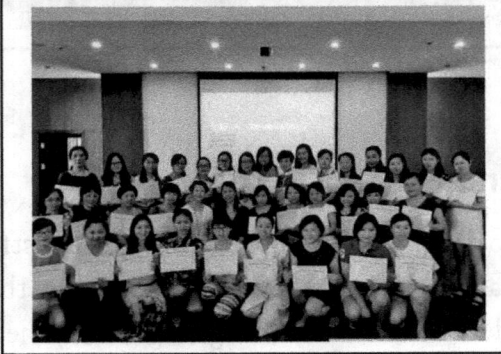

Figure 6. Training class in Shanghai for aspiring IBCLCs. Liz, front row, fourth from left.

At the second training for the medical staff, the chief of medicine presented me with an academic appointment: Outpatient Expert for International Medical Care—Postpartum Depression Care. We had a long talk about acupuncture. She was surprised, and rather pleased, that I knew about it. When I started talking about meridian points, she was convinced. She was happy to hear that it could be a treatment for depression because she thought it would be more acceptable for her patients.

Pre- and Postnatal Classes

I also taught six classes for new and expecting parents (Figure 7). I realized fairly quickly that my normal slides on depression and breastfeeding were far too academic for these groups of parents. So what I started doing was presenting for 15 to 30 minutes and then pulling up a chair and offering to answer their questions. In every class, we had more than an hour and a half of questions. The parents asked about breastfeeding, sleep, labor, and stress postpartum. I answered lots of basic breast-feeding questions, often using my fist to represent the breast and my other hand to represent the baby's mouth. That always made the mothers and fathers laugh. (I stopped using my other visual aids once I realized there were dads in the classes.)

Figure 7. Parents in a prenatal class, many expecting their second babies.

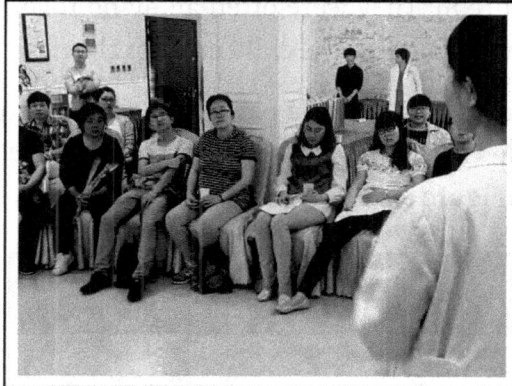

I taught basic breast massage and breast compression. Many also reported that their babies were falling asleep quickly at the breast. We talked about possibly removing some of the babies' clothing while nursing. Babies are often quite bundled up, even when it's warm outside, because Chinese mothers, and their mothers, are worried that babies (and new mothers)

will get cold. I mentioned that having a lot of clothing on could be making their babies sleepy. The conference room was typically more than 90°F.

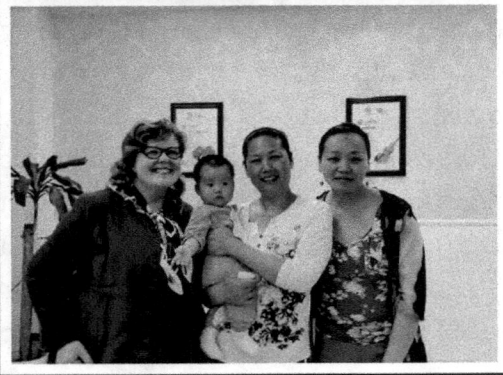

Figure 8. A new mother with her daughter and mother.

Grandmothers often came to the class with the mothers and fathers (Figure 8). They were often all living together. Grandparents provide much of the child care for the new babies.

The hospital also hosts a party for women who are newly postpartum. They come in their pajamas and are served an elegant tea (Figure 9).

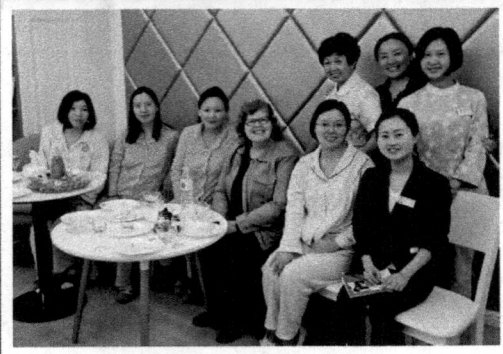

Figure 9. At the postpartum tea with a group of mothers still in the hospital.

International Day of the Nurse

On my final night, I was invited to join the nurses for their dinner for International Day of the Nurse (Figures 10 & 11). Dinner was placed on a large lazy Susan and we all helped ourselves with chopsticks right off the serving dishes. The hospital CEO and nursing director came around to each table. There were multiple toasts throughout the evening. My translator warned me to not empty my glass because it was a tradition in China to keep refilling your glass. Soon you've had way more to drink than you intended.

At the dinner, the hospital CEO presented me with a beautiful scarf made with Hangzhou silk. He told me that based on my visit, they decided to hire a psychologist to help new mothers with depression. I was quite happy about that. I was also happy that I had a chance to meet such warm and lovely people. I have promised that I would return. We are all still in touch.

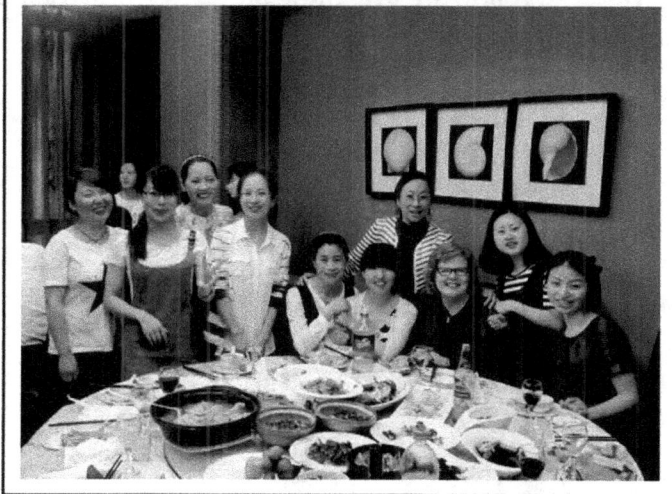

Figure 10. With some of the nurses at International Day of the Nurse celebration.

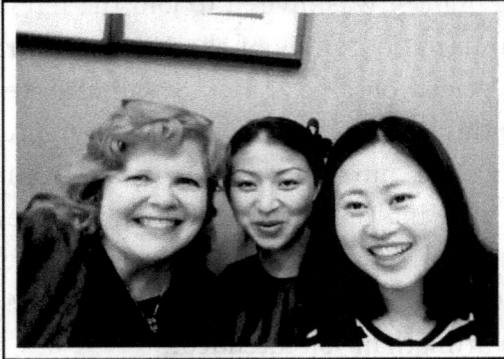

Figure 11. With midwife, Liz Jiang, and my translator, Alisa Hu.

The following text is a bit more about this beautiful city. It's no surprise that it is a popular place to go.

Some of the Sites That Make Hangzhou a Tourist Destination

Hangzhou does a brisk business in tourism. Even on a weekday, in the middle of the day, there were huge crowds of people. West Lake is a major attraction in Hangzhou, and it is easy to see why. The following are a few pictures from West Lake (Figures 12–15).

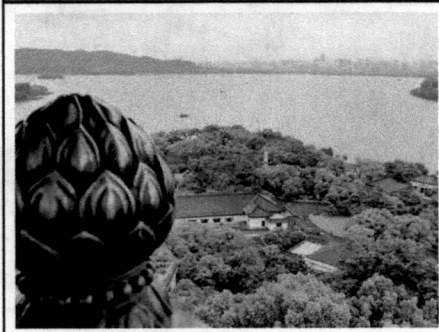

Figure 12. From the top of the Lingyin Temple with view of West Lake and the city in the background.

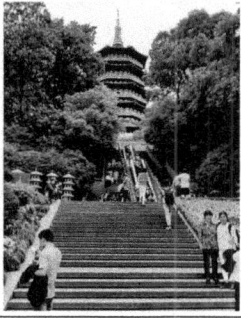

Figure 13. Lingyin Temple, with escalators that go up, but none that go down.

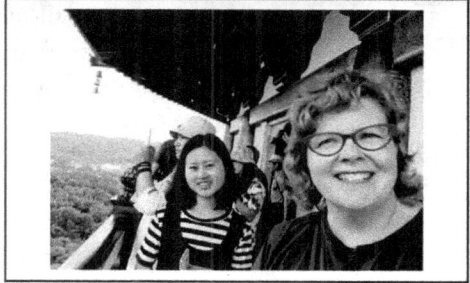

Figure 14. With my translator Alisa at the Lingyin Temple.

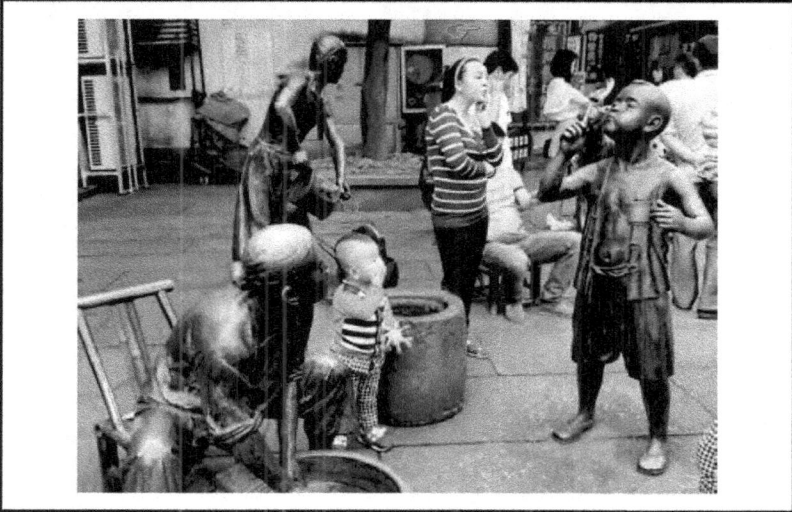

Figure 15. One of many babies we saw, this one was enjoying the statues in the West Lake Shopping District.

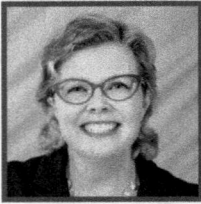

Kathleen Kendall-Tackett, PhD, IBCLC, RLC, FAPA, is a health psychologist, IBCLC, and the owner and editor-in-chief of Praeclarus Press, a small press specializing in women's health. Dr. Kendall-Tackett is editor-in-chief of two peer-reviewed journals, Clinical Lactation and Psychological Trauma. She is a fellow of the American Psychological Association in Health and Trauma Psychology and past president of the American Psychological Association Division of Trauma Psychology. Dr. Kendall-Tackett specializes in women's health research including breastfeeding, depression, trauma, and health psychology. Her research interests include the psychoneuroimmunology of maternal depression and the lifetime health effects of trauma.

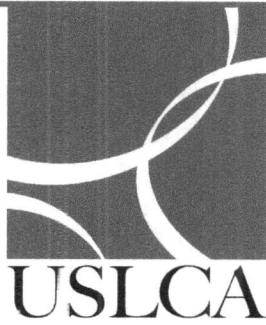

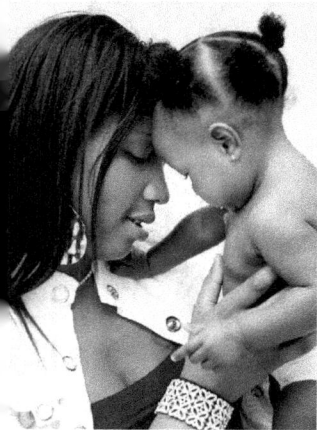

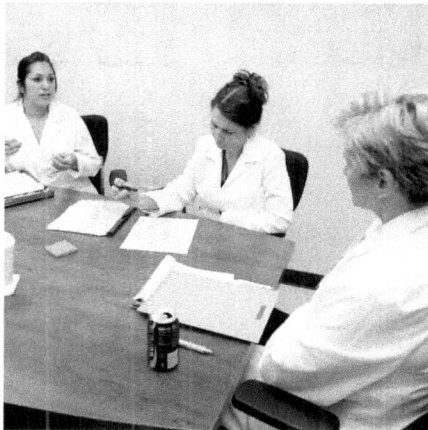

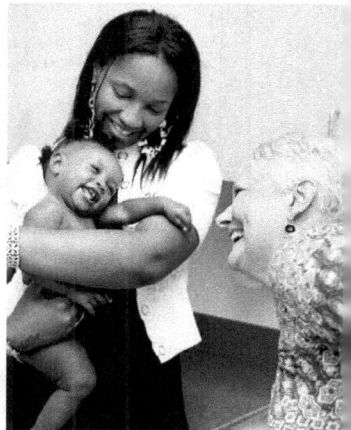

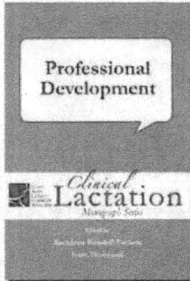

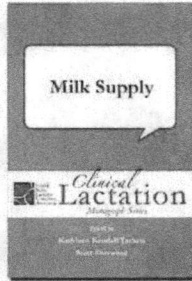

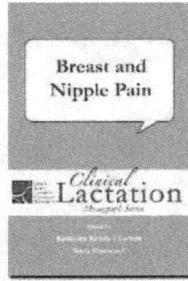

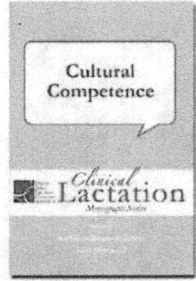

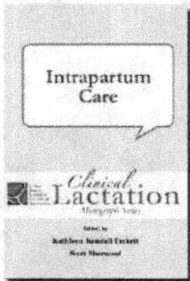

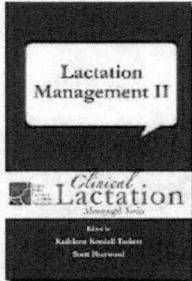

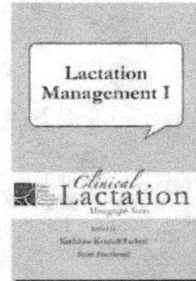

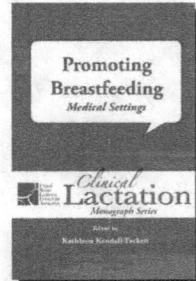

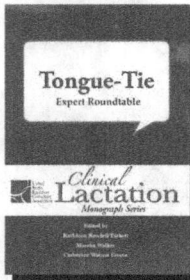

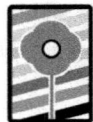

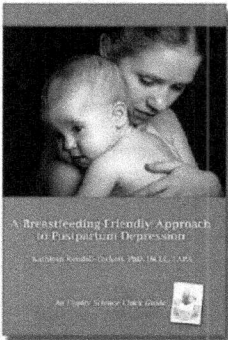

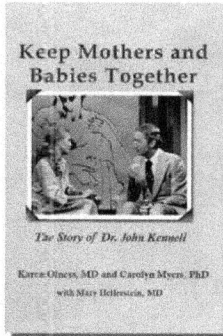

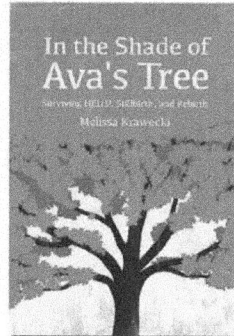

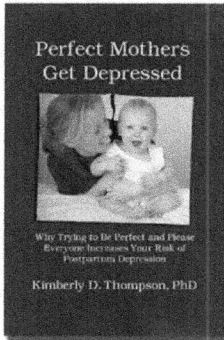

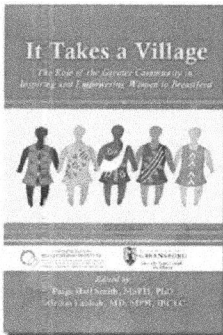

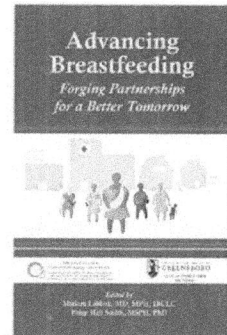

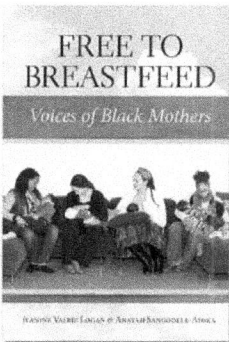

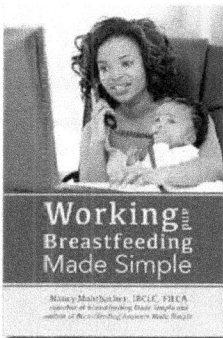

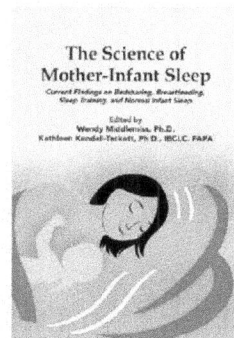

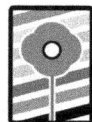